The Real Life
of a Pediatrician

D0871690

The Real Life of a Pediatrician

Perri Klass, MD

EDITOR

KAPLAN PUBLISHING

© 2009 Kaplan, Inc.

Published by Kaplan Publishing, a division of Kaplan, Inc.
1 Liberty Plaza, 24th Floor
New York, NY 10006

Printed in the United States

Real life of a pediatrician / Perri Klass, editor.
     p. ; cm. -- (Kaplan voices)
   ISBN 978-1-4277-9963-0 (pbk.)
   1. Pediatrics--Personnal narratives. 2. Pediatricians--Personnal narratives.
   I. Klass, Perri, 1958- II. Series: Kaplan voices.
   [DNLM: 1. Pediatrics--Personal Narratives. 2. Physicians--Personal
   Narratives. WS 21 R288 2009]
   RJ43.A1R43 2009
   618.92--dc22

                                          2009001491

10 9 8 7 6 5 4 3 2 1

ISBN-13: 978-1-4277-9963-0

CONTENTS

———

INTRODUCTION

Perri Klass, MD

PEDIATRICIANS HAVE GOOD stories to tell. The essence of pediatrics involves the most remarkable and most basic human story: the growth and change that takes each of us from newborn infant to child to adolescent to young adult. Every aspect of that growth and change informs at least some part of pediatrics; collectively, we pediatricians take as our professional property everyone from the premature newborn baby who weighs less than a pound to the high school football player who stands well over six feet tall and weighs in at more than 200 pounds. No other field in medicine includes patients separated along this logarithmic scale — the 1-kilogram baby (a premature infant weighing just over 2 pounds), the 10-kilogram child (22 pounds, a very nice weight for a toddler), and the 100-kilogram adolescent. It's our job, collectively, in pediatrics, to worry about the illnesses and injuries across all those ages and sizes.

Pediatrics is a relatively new field in medicine, dating back to the middle of the 19th century, and it is founded on the principle that, as they repeat over and over to us during our training, children are not small adults. Abraham Jacobi, the founding father of pediatrics, put it this way: "Pediatrics does not deal with miniature men and women, with reduced doses and the same class of diseases in smaller bodies. ...it has its own independent range and horizon and gives as much to general medicine as it receives from it." In the diseases and dangers that confront them, in their remarkable resilience but also in their vulnerabilities, in their responses to medications — in all of these ways, children are distinct and different, and their health care presents special challenges and conundrums.

As children are not small adults, it is also worth remembering that, as the World Health Organization puts it, health is more than the absence of disease. When you take care of children's health, you worry, of course, about preventing and treating illnesses and injuries and chronic diseases, but you also think constantly about how to foster and promote healthy development and everything that should come with it, from play and pleasure to learning and language.

We who practice pediatrics at this particular time and in the comparative luxury of a developed country are privileged to be practicing at a remarkable historical moment. Thanks to public health and hygiene, and especially to vaccines, we can watch our patients grow up free of many of the dangers that all through history have caused infant and child mortality — and that still hurt and kill children in many parts of the world. As recently as my own parents' generation, doctors — and mothers and fathers — had to worry about polio, about measles and rubella, about infection and paralysis and brain damage and death. My own oldest child was not protected as an infant against bacterial meningitis because the HIB vaccine only came along in time for his younger sister; as a resident, I took care of children with meningitis and worried that there was no way to protect my own son. The conquest of the vaccine-preventable infectious diseases doesn't mean that parents can stop worrying, of course, or that pediatricians can stop worrying. Part of the job of child rearing involves worrying about the safety and well-being of each and every profoundly beloved and profoundly vulnerable baby — and part of the job of pediatrics involves appreciating that the parents have in turn entrusted you with that baby, that child, even that teenager.

A newborn baby is a pediatric patient — and in fact, everyone begins the career of being a pediatric patient as a newborn baby. However, there is not a single newborn baby anywhere who has ever come in alone to see the doctor — every pediatric patient comes in the context of a family, brought in by parents, grandparents, or other caregivers. And part of the great privilege of practicing pediatrics is the sense of being woven into many lives, many families, and many stories. For pediatricians, that means being included over and over in those moments of astonished recognition that happen as children grow: yes, this rambunctious 5-year-old was that tiny, helpless baby; yes, that self-conscious, gangly 12-year-old has become this gracious young adult. I find myself identifying over and over with parents in their pride and their delight and, of course, in their anxiety — and sometimes in their grief.

It's also our role to see our patients through the age of pediatric expertise and then say good-bye to them as they grow into adulthood. Put simply, one great job — and one great joy — of pediatrics is watching our patients outgrow us; our goal is to shepherd them safely through childhood and into adulthood, and then pass them on to other doctors who will worry about the medical issues of those grown-up years. And this is true in every area of pediatrics, including pediatric oncology and neurosurgery — we all want to see our patients outgrow and outlive our period of expertise. It isn't at all true in adult medicine, which necessarily and properly includes the end of every patient's lifespan as part of the territory. In pediatrics, we want our patients to grow up and leave us behind.

Medical careers reflect their own trajectories of growth and change, and there are stories here that describe the different developmental stages of a life in pediatrics. William Borkowsky looks back on the conversations and decisions that took him into the field of pediatrics and talks about the influence that teachers and mentors can have. Bryan Vartabedian finds himself thinking about how he can best play that same role for a young student, by example and by advice.

Medical training involves so many stages of increasing

knowledge and increasing responsibility. Alenka Zeman tells the story of finding herself in charge of a terrifyingly ill child. As a resident, covering at a community hospital, she must take care of a child who may be about to die; the child's grandparents are looking to her to handle the situation. It's overwhelming, it's frightening, it's impossible — and it's her job. Michael Patrick tells another story out of training, in which an intern picks up a chart in the emergency room and finds himself caring for a dangerously ill child and trying to reassure the mother.

There are essays here that reflect a tremendous variety of locations and situations, all of them places where children are growing up and pediatricians are caring for them. Stacy Stryer describes a rather unusual training situation as she gets ready to practice on a remote Navajo reservation; Lee Beers describes practicing on a military base in Guantánamo Bay. But whether the pediatrician is Joy Neyhart in Alaska or Rachel Kowalsky in a New York City emergency room, the connections to individual children and individual families are paramount, and these essays are also about trying to understand the story and the circumstances of a particular family.

The great joy of primary care pediatrics is the opportunity to work with families over time and to understand their stories; some of the essays in this collection show us those long-term relationships between a pediatrician and a family, or even a pediatrician and a community of families. In doing so, the authors reflect on the different kinds of lessons that they have learned from these relationships. Mariana Glusman recounts her many years of caring for a child and her changing understanding of that child and her mother. Diego Chaves-Gnecco describes a longtime relationship with a single child that reflects his own journey with an entire community of Spanish-speaking families. Christine Gleason describes the joy of claiming a new baby as a primary care patient — and then the unexpected changes in the relationship over time.

Working with families over time means developing relationships that change as the children grow and can often become complex and nuanced; Eileen Costello discusses some of the delicate situations that arise when a pediatrician is placed uncomfortably in the middle between a parent and a child. It's part of our job to help them understand one another, and sometimes we find ourselves trying to help them connect.

As I said above, in pediatrics we expect our patients to survive their illnesses and, indeed, to outgrow the pediatric phase of life. Perhaps for this reason, several of the writers in this collection find themselves looking back on those children who did not survive and on their own reactions. Dipesh Navsaria talks about trying to find and understand the proper role to play when a baby dies, and about the terrible power such a death has over all the people caring for that baby in a newborn intensive care unit. Suzanne Dixon reflects on similar questions in a very different setting when she describes her experiences in rural Kenya with a child who does not survive.

Certain themes come up again and again when pediatricians discuss our job, tell our stories, or write them down. There is that idea of overwhelming responsibility — that people should trust us with their children and look to us when their children are sick. There is the notion of understanding very different families, different cultures, and different child-rearing practices so that we can help parents with something as basic as how to feed a baby. There is also always the shadow that hangs over pediatrics; not all parents are competent, and not all children are properly cared for. In Rachel Kowalsky's essay about a family in the emergency room suspected of child abuse, or in my own story of reporting a mother to the authorities and wondering whether I have helped her or harmed her, we confront the professional imperative that we keep an eye out, always, for abuse and neglect and the things that can complicate our relationships with parents.

Many writers touch on the themes of how doctors learn to understand their patients, whether that means decoding an unfamiliar cultural context or assimilating new life experiences that enlarge their perspective. Thus, Huy Nguyen writes about trying to understand the beliefs and practices and the history and customs that are getting in the way of a Vietnamese baby's growth and finds wisdom in a Vietnamese proverb: "To appreciate me, you must appreciate the road I have taken to come here." Patrick McDonald learns to explain — and to understand — neurosurgical care in terms that make sense to a First Nations family in Winnipeg. Diego Chaves-Gnecco learns from his patient how to understand "my role as a pediatrician in our community, the Latino pediatrician who is part of the community he serves, who goes to church with his patients."

We learn from our patients, but we also learn from the changes in our own lives. Lee Beers describes the impact that her own pregnancies and miscarriages have had on her understanding of parents; Sayantani DasGupta draws connections between her own experience as a patient undergoing a medical procedure and the procedures she has performed on children.

Most of all, however, these essays return again and again to the joys and the sorrows of being part of children's lives and families' lives in all the many different settings in which pediatricians practice. We learn from our patients, we learn from their families, we learn from our own mistakes and victories as the children grow and change and develop and as the doctor's story and the patients' stories connect and branch and echo and intertwine.

Baptism by Fire

Alenka Zeman, MD

I FELT THAT THERE was something different about that
bleak day even before it started. I woke up before the
sun had a chance to rise and drove in the cold winter
morning to the community hospital where I was spending
a month as the supervising resident. A trip that normally
took close to an hour on those slippery winter mornings
took me only 30 minutes this time. For some reason, there
were no traffic jams, breakdowns, or ice between me and
the hospital. In hindsight, it feels as though fate was beck-
oning me to the hospital.

As an overworked resident, my first emotion when I
stepped into the hospital that morning was frustration. "I
could still be in bed," I muttered to myself as the glass front

doors to the hospital creaked open. The cafeteria was not even open yet, so I couldn't grab a cup of coffee. Lacking sufficient caffeine, I shuffled upstairs and plopped myself in front of a computer, hoping that I would be invisible for 30 minutes until I could get a sign-out report on the patients from the overnight doctor.

I hoped I would have a brief respite, but a little later, I heard my intern (a first-year resident) storm into the room. "Wow," I thought. "She's here early too." Her voice was hesitant as she struggled to get my attention. "There was a kid admitted last night with gastroenteritis." I barely looked up from my computer.

Gastroenteritis is a viral illness that causes vomiting and diarrhea. It swarms the pediatric floors during the winter and is one of the most common illnesses we take care of as residents. In fact, we consider it a rite of passage to come down with profuse diarrhea before we graduate. So of course, it wasn't out of the ordinary to see an admission with that diagnosis at this time of year. "Do you think you could come take a look at him?" she asked. "He has this funny breathing pattern, as if he has diabetes." The intern's voice grew more urgent, but what she was saying was inconsistent with the normal blood sugar level I had seen on the computer lab list for this patient. I looked up from the computer and was about to explain to her that there was no way this child had diabetes, when I saw the worried look on her face. I knew then that I had to go and see the child for myself.

I will never forget the feeling in my chest when

I walked into that child's room with my intern trailing behind me. It was dark, but in the distant corner I could see a large metal crib with tall hospital rails on the side. Inside the crib was a very thin two-year-old child with floppy blond hair lying rigid and flat on his back. His arms were straight at his side and he kept extending them in an odd, repetitive motion. This was something I had been taught to recognize in medical school but had never seen in real life. It was a situation that I had hoped I would never see, because it meant that he was posturing from swelling in his brain. As I entered the room I had expected to see a mother or father at the bedside. Instead, I saw an older man and woman, likely the grandparents, sitting in the corner with a four-year-old sibling draped on their knees. The grandmother whispered, "Please don't disturb him. He is finally sleeping peacefully."

My heart sank again, because I realized I didn't even know this child's first name. I had never met these people before, and now somehow, in a matter of seconds, I had to express to them that their grandchild was very sick, that he could die, and that they needed to trust me. But why should they trust me? I didn't know much, if anything, about their grandchild outside of the dire situation that he was in. I was only in my second year of pediatric residency, but one of the big lessons we learn early on is to recognize sick children versus not-sick children. At the time, I wasn't sure how I was going to help this child, but I knew I had to do something fast—or he was going to die.

I ran to the side of the crib and used all my strength

to lower those creaky iron rails that flanked it. I picked up the child, and his weak, exhausted body just sank into my arms. I left my intern to explain to the grandparents what was happening and rushed with the child to the treatment room, where I could gather nurses and equipment. I was unable to make eye contact with the family as I left the room. Maybe I didn't want to see their scared faces, or perhaps I did not want them to see how petrified I was.

Acute cerebral herniation, or brain swelling, is something that we all learn how to manage in medical school — but it is rarely something that you deal with in real life unless you have chosen to become a brain surgeon. It is definitely rarely encountered in a small community hospital like the one where I, as a second-year resident, was the doctor in charge. When I chose pediatrics as a career, I was hoping that I would never have to deal with acute neurological emergencies like this, but there was no avoiding it now.

The next 15 minutes felt like an out-of-body experience. I stood at the head of the bed calling out orders, but my mind kept fixating on the fact that a child's life was in my hands. I could hear myself calling a "Code Blue," which signified that this child was dangerously close to death and that I needed help. The room began to fill with nurses and other doctors who were ready to help out. Everyone started falling into his or her role: the anesthesiologists were putting a tube down the patient's throat to help him breathe; one nurse was drawing blood and starting more lines in the patient; another nurse was pushing the medications to try to stop his brain from swelling; and a handful of other assistants were hustling in and out of the room, bringing more supplies. Even the medical students were standing at attention in the corner, ready to help out if something was needed. I seemed to be calling out orders one by one, but I couldn't even follow what I was saying, as my heart and brain both seemed to be racing at warp speed.

My intern thrust a cell phone to my ear, and fortunately, there was a very calming voice on the other end. "I know you can do this. We have talked about what to do in this situation," the voice said. It was the pediatric intensive care unit fellow in my own hospital, the major hospital about 45 minutes away in the center of the city. "Just get him stabilized. I am mobilizing the flight team to come pick him up." Of course, I knew that if I were sitting in the middle of a lecture at the hospital, calmly sipping a cup of coffee, I would be able to quickly recount the steps a resident would need to go through in this situation. None of my training had prepared me for how I would feel when I saw a young child unresponsive because of the acute changes in his brain.

Out of the corner of my eye, I saw a figure dressed in black approach the doorway. I turned and saw the child's grandfather, with tears cascading over the wrinkles in his face. He was leaning on the shoulder of a priest as they tiptoed into the room together. "My grandchild has never been baptized. I need for him to be baptized…just in case." There was no question that the grandfather understood the seriousness of this moment. I silently nodded, and the sea of nursing staff parted for the priest and grandfather to slip to the head of the bed. Drops of water splattered on the child's forehead, and a sense of tranquility filled the room as everyone stopped for a few seconds to watch the ceremony. The priest uttered the child's name for the first time: "Timothy."

The moment of silence was interrupted by a booming voice announcing that the CT scanner was ready. We needed to wheel the child downstairs for imaging so that we could better understand why his brain had swelled so suddenly. I gently peeled the grandfather's fingers off his grandchild. "We need to go now, but I promise he will be in good hands," I whispered softly. The grandfather and I made eye contact for the first time.He did not speak, but with his silent nod, I knew he was trusting me to take care of his grandchild.

When the image appeared on the monitor next to the CT scanner, there was no need for the radiologist to explain to the crowd what we saw. There was a huge mass in the posterior aspect of the brain. A brain tumor. The story started to fall into place. My intern had by then contacted the child's parents, who were away on vacation, and they had reported that he would throw up every morning. This had caused him to lose a significant amount of weight. The grandparents had come to visit, noticed these symptoms, and thus wisely brought him to the hospital to be evaluated. Every pediatrician fears that a case of vomiting will be dismissed as a mere virus when in reality the child has an undiagnosed brain tumor. In fact, this is a very rare turn of events, but Timothy's case was one of those exceptions.

The door opened, and four people in bright blue flight suits with red backpacks appeared. In a morning that had already been filled with religious moments, I couldn't help thinking that angels had arrived. The med flight team was here. They quickly and efficiently assumed the care of the child, loaded him on the stretcher, and whisked him off to the helicopter. I knew that in about ten minutes, Timothy would be landing on the roof of the intensive care unit, where a crew of neurosurgeons would be waiting eagerly to assume his care.

After the child was safely en route to the bigger hospital, the doctors and nurses in the treatment room were gone just as quickly as they had arrived. Before I knew it, I was standing by an empty stretcher in a room littered with supplies, with nothing but my thoughts to keep me company. What if the grandparents had not brought him in to the hospital the night before? He probably would have died at home in his sleep. What if the traffic patterns had changed and my intern had not been here to check on him early in the morning? And now, what will his overall prognosis be?

I leaned my head on the stretcher, and the tears that I had been holding back all morning came flowing out. I wasn't sure whether they were tears of sadness, relief, or even joy because I could actually say that I had saved the life of a child. All I knew was that it felt good to release some of my pent-up emotions. As I wiped off my face, I knew that I had to get back to caring for the other 15 children on the floor. And the team would be waiting for me to discuss what had happened. I exited the room, but before I left, I looked back to the spot where I had seen a child baptized and realized that I, too, had been baptized — by fire.

THIRSTY

Michael Patrick, MD

AN INTERN'S LIFE in the pediatric emergency department isn't exactly what you'd call exciting. You see lots of colds and scrapes and ear infections. The interesting problems — such as asthma, diabetes, and broken bones — are gobbled up by the junior and senior residents.

So you can imagine my excitement late one night toward the end of my intern year when I looked up at the big write-on wipe-off board and saw a name written in black marker. Not green. Not blue or red. But black, the color code for the most serious cases in the ER. These kids weren't for interns, unless the doc in charge of the department, the attending physician, gave us special permission.

A resident should have taken the case, but they were all occupied with other kids. My gaze turned from the board to the attending. Then back to the board. Then back to the attending. This time our eyes met, and he responded with a nod and a smile.

Without an ounce of hesitation, I hurried to the rack and picked up the chart. "You coming with me?" I asked.

"No," he said. "You can do it alone."

Really? He'd let me see this one alone? I guess it made sense. In a couple of months I'd be a junior resident, and then there'd be no choice — I'd have to see kids like this alone. At least this way, if I messed up, I could still play the intern card.

Well, as it turns out, I didn't mess up…at least not in the traditional sense.

I WALKED INTO the examination room and introduced myself to the boy's mother. Black mascara ran down her cheeks, which seemed odd. I could understand the display of emotion had the boy been strapped to a backboard with a rigid cervical collar around his neck, or if he'd been gasping for air and wheezing to beat the band. But as it turned out, the carrot-topped, freckle-faced two-year-old sat on the edge of the bed swinging his legs.

I looked around the room for a critically ill patient. But aside from me, the mom, and the boy, the room was empty.

"Is this James?" I asked.

Between sobs, the mom confirmed that it was.

"And he's thirsty," she added. "My little Jimmy is really, really thirsty."

I looked over at the boy. "Are you thirsty?"

He nodded. "Yes, Mister. You gots lemonade?"

The mom began to lose it all over again. Her voice cracked with slow and deliberate words. "That's his problem, doctor. All he does is drink and pee. Drink and pee. Drink and pee. That's it. Then tonight he starts puking. So I took him to St. Anne's Hospital. You know the one…across town. They did some tests and said his sugar's really, really high."

She paused, her eyes producing fresh tears. Then she started in again, this time faster and through a new round of sobs, "He has diabetes, doctor! They said my little Jimmy has diabetes! And they said they can't do a damn thing for him…except send him here."

She looked at me with one of those looks you never forget. "But you can help him. Right, doctor? Tell me you can help him!"

"I want lemonade! Mister, you gots lemonade or what?"

Mom regrouped. "He's not a Mister, Jimmy. He's a doctor. And I told you before…you can't have lemonade." Then suddenly, through the greatest sob yet, "Lemonade's got sugar!"

"But I want lemonade! Doctor, please! Gets me lemonade!"

His mom was falling apart, and I knew little Jimmy would fall apart too if she kept this up.

"Let's take a look at you, Jimmy. Then we'll see if we can't find you a glass of lemonade."

"Really?" he asked.

"Really," I said. "Because I know you're thirsty."

I FINISHED MY physical examination and studied the lab data from the referring hospital. The situation was clear: little Jimmy was extremely dehydrated. He needed IV fluids and he needed them fast. His blood pressure was fine, but his heart was racing. Diabetic ketoacidosis with compensated hypovolemic shock. I'd read about it and answered test questions on the subject, but this was my first experience up close and personal. And what surprised me the most was just how good the kid looked — sitting up, smiling, kicking his legs, and begging for a glass of lemonade.

I discussed the case with the ER attending, and soon little Jimmy had IV fluids, insulin, more blood work pending, and a hospital bed in the intensive care unit. I even found him a glass of diet lemonade for sipping, thanks to the dietary department and their stock of diabetes-friendly beverages.

Soon the ICU residents would be down to do their history and physical. After that, little Jimmy would go to the unit, and I would move on to my next patient.

I WAS FEELING pretty good. Sure, I was just an intern, but I had really nailed this one. I'd figured out the right amount of fluids and the correct dose of insulin, ordered the necessary labs, and called the intensive care unit and endocrine attendings to present the case for admission.

Before picking up a new chart, I thought I'd pop my head in the door and see if little Jimmy or his mom needed anything. By this time, his mom was remarkably composed, and I'll take credit for her recovery. I've always enjoyed the fine art of patient/parent education, and my thorough explanation of diabetes and detailed description of little Jimmy's course over the next few days went a long way toward demystifying her son's condition.

Of course, I didn't tell her everything. Life-threatening complications can arise with new-onset diabetics. In fact, they always go to the intensive care unit that first night—just in case. But the truth is those complications almost never happen. And with the mom upset anyway, I thought it best to keep those details to myself.

The arrival of a couple of family members also helped. And then there was little Jimmy. He had turned out to be a real trooper, taking the IV stick in stride and busying himself with the Disney Channel on his bedside TV.

The mom's makeup streaks were gone now, and she actually had a smile on her face when I walked in the room.

One of the newcomers spoke first. "Are you sure he's okay, Doctor?"

Mom's smile disappeared.

I put a reassuring hand on little Jimmy's leg and repeated the highlights of my earlier spiel.

"Well, it's going to be a life change, that's for sure. He'll need daily shots of insulin and frequent monitoring of his blood sugar. But look, lots of kids have diabetes and live happy lives. Believe me, there are worse conditions out there!"

I saw the smile slowly return, and I imagined Mom going over in her head the details we had discussed before. Knowledge erases fear, and I knew I had done a good job explaining this thing.

"Of course, there will be difficult moments," I continued. "He won't want the injections at first, but he'll get used to them. And they're working on new technologies like crazy—insulin pumps, a nose-spray version, even an artificial pancreas."

"But what about tonight?" It was the other relative. "Will he be okay tonight? If the future's so bright, why are you sending him to the intensive care unit? That seems pretty extreme to me."

Mom's smile disappeared again, and I sensed this wasn't the time to describe the possible (but highly unlikely) complications associated with new-onset diabetes.

"Well…we have to lower his blood sugar slowly. That means he'll need hourly blood draws to watch his serum glucose. That's too much work for the regular floor. The ICU is better staffed to get those done on time."

The stranger accepted this answer, but Mom didn't look convinced. In fact, those three letters seemed to erase all my reassurance.

"I-C-U," she repeated, her voice faint and far away. "He really has to go to the ICU?"

As if on cue, the admitting team arrived to do their workup, and I excused myself. But I didn't go far. I wanted to say a final good-bye before they rolled little Jimmy upstairs.

THE NEXT MORNING, I left home early so I could swing by the pediatric ICU and visit little Jimmy and his mom. This was new territory for me. I guess it's because you don't really get a chance to form a bond with patients and parents in the fast and furious world of emergency medicine. Faces and problems come and go like cards in a casino. But I wanted to see how Mom was holding up. I wanted to say, "See, I told you everything would be all right."

Unfortunately, I hit bad traffic and arrived at the hospital five minutes after the start of my shift. Still, I didn't think the ER attending would mind me being late once I explained the reason, so I bypassed the emergency department and went upstairs.

I hurried through the automatic doors leading into the ICU and scanned their version of the big write-on wipe-off board, looking for little Jimmy's name.

It wasn't there.

I glanced around the dimly lit unit, figuring one of the residents could give me an update and point me in the right direction. I assumed little Jimmy's blood sugar had come down without a hitch, and the ICU docs had already transferred him to the endocrine floor.

Unfortunately, the house staff were knee deep in rounds. The unit clerk was knee deep too, arguing on the phone with the pharmacy about a delayed drug delivery. And, of course, the nurses were all busy with the myriad of activities it takes to keep chaos from raining down upon an intensive care unit.

I glanced at my watch. Five minutes late had turned into ten. Okay, I could swing through the endocrine ward on my way to the ER. I couldn't stay long, but I could say a quick hello. Then, after my shift, I'd return for a longer visit — to see how little Jimmy and his mom were holding up.

Except I couldn't find his name on their write-on wipe-off board either. The unit clerk for endocrine wasn't busy, so I asked whether she knew anything about an earlier transfer from the ICU.

The transfer didn't ring a bell, but she offered to look in the computer. Maybe he went to a different floor, although neither of us could think of a good reason for that — all the new-onset diabetics went to endocrine after discharge from the ICU.

Because of my growing tardiness, I declined the offer. I'd have to settle for looking on the computer myself…if I found a free moment during my shift.

I KNEW SOMETHING was wrong right away. The ER was in the midst of one of those unusual lulls, and everyone — residents, nurses, medical students, even the attending — was sitting around the nurse's station talking.

But when I joined the crowd, all chatter stopped, and everyone looked my way.

Through a nervous chuckle, I said, "Okay, so I'm late. I have a good reason."

The attending shook his head. "Don't worry about it. We're not busy. In fact, why don't you go down and watch the autopsy. Pathology just called with a couple questions. Apparently, they're ready to start."

I scrunched my brow. "What autopsy?"

"You haven't heard? That kid you saw yesterday. The new-onset diabetic. He died last night."

My eyes widened. "What…? You're kidding me, right?"

The ER vanished. My mind raced. I had promised everything would be okay. I'd said worse things happen to kids, but what's worse than dead? I wanted to disappear. I wanted to go back to bed and start the day over. No, I wanted to go back to bed and start yesterday over. Forget about the interesting case. I would be perfectly happy with a green or blue or red chart.

But, of course, there are no do-overs in medicine, so I went downstairs and watched.

LITTLE JIMMY WAS the victim of a complication called cerebral edema. The simple story goes like this: As blood sugar falls, fluid has a tendency to leak out of blood vessels and move into tissues and organs through a process called osmosis. If lots of osmosis happens rapidly around the brain, then the brain swells, and since the brain is surrounded by solid bone, the swollen tissue has nowhere to go.

Well, that's not entirely true. There's a hole in the base of the skull where the spinal cord meets the brain. The tremendous pressure squeezes the brain stem through the opening, squishing it like a sausage link, and since that part of the brain controls important things (such as breathing), it's a situation generally incompatible with life.

Cerebral edema is a rare complication in diabetics, and until I met little Jimmy, I had never seen it. In the 13 years since that meeting, I've never seen it again. Not once.

Was I wrong to give his mom reassurance? Did it amount to false hope? For a long time, I thought so. For a long time, I was stingy in the reassurance department. I described every possible risk in lurid detail, even when the risk was minuscule. As a result, I scared the bajabbers out of many parents.

I have softened with time. Reassurance comes easier these days — although it's always qualified. Instead of saying, "Everything will be fine," I say, "Chances are really, really good that everything will be fine."

Even after all this time, it's the best I can do.

I never saw little Jimmy's mother again. Did she blame me for setting her up for a horrific fall? Maybe. I'll never know. But I do know this: Little Jimmy wasn't the only one thirsty that night. His mom was thirsty too. Thirsty for reassurance. And me? I guess I was young, I was much too confident, and I was thirsty to provide it.

My Mentor Was a Swine

Stacy Beller Stryer, MD

As physicians, we all have our mentors who have taught us the lessons we carry throughout our professional careers. Personally, I have had several memorable teachers — one of them just happened to come in the form of a hog.

I met my mentor in the summer of 1997. Earlier that same season, my husband, an internist, and I, a pediatrician, had just signed on to work for the Indian Health Service. We had decided to work in Kayenta, a small town on the Navajo reservation in northern Arizona. Kayenta was in the middle of nowhere, without a single traffic light, and the closest Target and Wal-Mart were two and a half hours away. Yet we were very excited to be moving there.

Not only were we going to have the opportunity to see a new part of the country, but we were also going to learn about a culture where the language and customs were very different from our own.

Although I was thrilled to begin my new job, I was also pretty nervous. While working at the Kayenta health clinic, we would be expected to be full-service docs, responsible for treating everyone and everything. Of course I would be taking care of children, which was great. However, I would also be treating adults in the clinics and in the emergency room. That wasn't so great. I had not treated someone with vascular disease or an actual heart attack since my medical school days. And I had certainly never been the physician solely responsible for treating someone who had been in an accident and needed emergency, life-or-death care. I was about to embark on a journey where all of these situations were not only possible but probable, and I had to be prepared. I could no longer call on my attending or quickly transfer a patient to the intensive care unit. I *was* the attending. And I *was* the intensive care unit. To make things even scarier, the closest hospital was in Tuba City, a mere 73 miles away.

Luckily, the administration within the Indian Health Service was aware of how rusty we all were when it came to seeing patients outside our own specialty, so they scheduled several refresher and training courses to bring us up to speed. After we arrived, I, my husband, and about five other new physicians were whisked from training session to training session. First we recertified in basic cardiopulmonary resuscitation (CPR), where we were reminded how to evaluate and help someone who was not breathing and had no heart rate. Then we renewed our certifications in Pediatric Advanced Life Support (PALS). I laughed when the internists shook in fear at the sight of the tiny baby mannequins. They seemed afraid even to touch the plastic dolls. But it was their turn to laugh at me and the other pediatricians during Advanced Cardiac Life Support training, when we had to evaluate adults who were having chest pain or difficulty breathing.

After we all felt comfortable evaluating infants who weren't breathing and adults who were clutching their chests, we carpooled to intensely hot Phoenix, Arizona, five hours away. We, and other new Indian Health Service physicians, were about to embark on two days of sheer terror as we trained in Advanced Trauma Lifesaving. The idea of the trauma is what frightened me the most. I knew that this meant I might encounter someone who had been severely injured in a car accident, in a fight, or by a bull during a rodeo. Unfortunately, all of these were distinct possibilities. I knew that the rate of car accidents was much greater on the reservation, or "rez," probably due to a combination of factors, including increased alcohol intoxication, single-lane roads, poor lighting along those roads, and roaming animals.

During the first day of class I had trouble concentrating, because I knew what was coming next. The second day, we all walked into the makeshift emergency room. And that is when I met the hog. He and eleven of his friends were anesthetized and laid out on cold, metal tables. They had breathing tubes in their mouths, and their front legs were gently tied above their faces to allow access to their bodies. Although I could handle human traumas without a blink of an eye, the sight of the anesthetized hog immediately nauseated me. I began to sweat, and suddenly the room felt very hot. I calmed down and reminded myself that these hogs were here for our education — so that we could save people's lives.

We had been organized in groups so that each hog was surrounded by four to six physicians. Our instructors told us that we had to learn to treat three emergencies. The first was a hemopericardium, or blood filling the outside sac of the heart. The weight of the blood could keep the heart from pushing blood through the rest of the body, causing death. The second was a pneumothorax, or the collapse of one lung due to a variety of problems. The third was pleural effusion, or massive amounts of fluid in the lung. The treatments for these problems were, respectively, a needle inserted into the sac around the heart to remove the blood, a needle placed in the pleural cavity to remove extra air so the collapsed lung could reinflate, and a chest tube put into the lung to remove some of the fluid.

As you may have guessed, each of us needed to practice these procedures on our hog. Somehow I picked the short straw, so I had to go last. I watched and grew more anxious as each physician placed needles and tubes into the hog. I did notice, with relief, that the hog did not appear to be in any distress whatsoever. A heart monitor attached to my hog showed that his heart rate did not vary much from the baseline during the procedures. When it was finally my turn, I took a deep breath. I would place the chest tube first. I held the scalpel in my hand and concentrated very hard. I had to find the right place to put the tube so that I would not damage any nerves or injure any other organs. Yet there were several puncture wounds already on the skin from the other doctors' procedures.

I will never forget what happened next. As I bent down and put my first, hesitant nick in the skin, my hog suddenly whacked me on the back of my head with his front right leg. My heart rate and blood pressure shot through the roof as I screamed, and I jumped back as fast as I could. All the other physicians in the room immediately stopped what they were doing and stared at me. They began to laugh — and I think my husband laughed the hardest of all. It seemed that the rope that was holding the legs up had come undone. Gravity, along with perfect placement of my head, led to the surprise attack. After our instructor retied the hog's legs, I forced myself to stop shaking and calm down so that I could perform the three procedures.

Thankfully, the rest of the day was uneventful. However, I could not forget the incident. I returned to Kayenta and, when I was in the emergency room, frequently faced emergency situations. My hog had taught me some crucial lessons. For one, I learned how to force myself to stop shaking so I wouldn't make a mistake during the procedure or forget a critical step. I also learned how crucial it was, in general, to calm myself during very anxious times. I used this wisdom during a cardiac arrest, numerous heart attacks, and several horrendous car accidents. And today, I am still grateful that my hog knocked some sense into me so many years ago.

PATH TO PEDIATRICS

William Borkowsky, MD

WHAT IS A pediatrician, anyway?

Dr. Zimmerman, my childhood pediatrician, must have asked himself that question at one time, before he decided to enter and complete a pediatric residency in midlife after practicing general medicine for over a decade. A general practitioner, as one was called then, took care of children in addition to adults. Was he disenchanted with adults or particularly enamored with children? I never got to ask him that question. But his sacrifice meant one thing for me: his *Highlights* and *Humpty Dumpty* magazine-laden waiting room was a welcome change from the *Life* magazines I encountered in the waiting rooms of other physicians. If only he could order a *Superman* comic, too…

Most of my actual contact with Dr. Zimmerman was limited to an annual physical exam. My parents wouldn't allow me to be sick, and I usually complied with their wishes. Nevertheless, my true lasting impression of him came during a home visit, on a weekend when a fever and a pins-and-needles sensation swept through my body. He arrived, gave me an injection of penicillin, and assured me that I would recover unscathed. I was unfamiliar with illness, so it was comforting to know that it would retreat from my body, ensuring that I would miss no school.

I stopped seeing Dr. Zimmerman, and all other doctors, after becoming a high school student. I presume he thrived without me. But in the meantime, I became attracted to the concept of becoming a physician after reading Sinclair Lewis's *Arrowsmith* and watching Drs. Kildare and Casey on television. Since none of these doctors was a pediatrician, my knowledge of the specialty was not enhanced in any way.

By my third year of medical school, I was attracted to virtually every specialty, except psychiatry. Very few individuals hospitalized with psychiatric diseases left "cured" back then. Neither Freud nor thorazine was sufficiently active in this population to suit me. Pediatrics was interesting. Internal medicine was interesting. Surgery was interesting. A decision about my future would have to emerge in the coming months — and how would I come to it? If you ask pediatricians why they chose their field, a typical answer is, "I didn't want to see children suffering." If you ask internists why they *didn't* choose pediatrics, a typical answer is, "I didn't want to see children suffering." Clearly, empathy or sympathy would not serve me for this choice. How, then, was I to proceed?

I needed to decide which group, internists or pediatricians, I would like to spend my time with. Thus, I watched different groups of physicians as they came into a basement dining room in the old Bellevue Hospital. This large, cafeteria-style establishment was a potential escape area for interns and residents, hungry or not. The entrance was a door that pushed open into the chamber. Surgeons typically burst through the door, boldly marching in as a group. Woe to the poor individual already inside the dining room who reached for the door in order to get back to work! Many a hand or head was battered by the surgeons this way. The internal medicine residents also approached the swinging door as a group but in a more reticent manner. The door didn't burst open; it was carefully pushed so as not to injure anyone on the other side. But pediatricians often entered alone, with an approach to the door even more calculated than the internists'. They pushed the door open slowly to peer in and see whether there was anyone on the other side. Moreover, they would not simply let the door close behind them. Instead, the doctors would turn back to see that the door would not slam closed on the next person. Pediatricians were more caring! Obstetricians often waited for the door to open spontaneously, perhaps reflecting their medical approach to labor and delivery. The psychiatrists also approached the door alone, I should add, but often stopped short of opening the door, perhaps wondering whether they should go in at all. Hunger, after all, was but a state of mind.

Having settled what group of doctors I wanted to mingle with, I was leaning toward pediatrics but still somewhat drawn to the internists. At my medical school, there was an arrogance among the internists. Their specialty was the Queen of Medicine. Pediatricians were viewed as mere grown-up kids with medical degrees. Their "practice" was closer to "play" and did not require the intensity needed to treat seriously ill adults. Pediatricians did indeed "play" with sick children, but this seemed a plus to me rather than a minus. On the other hand, the critically ill, premature infants didn't play back. If play was a plus, "preemies" were a minus. Another minus was my difficulty in caring for adolescents. Their reactions to any attempts to educate and treat them were not unlike the reactions of the adult chronic alcoholic or drug addict. So I was still in a quandary.

By August of my fourth year of medical school, I needed to make a decision. Fortunately, fate intervened in an unexpected place. I had been spending my summers working in a children's summer camp in northeastern Pennsylvania for years, since graduating from high school. My chemistry teacher was responsible for recruiting waiters for this camp, and I must have looked like a potential recruit. When he first approached me about the camp, I had already been working full-time for the last two years of high school to earn money for college, and the pay for working in this camp for eight weeks was no more than I got in two weeks of my usual work schedule during the summer. I rejected the offer. Unrelenting, the teacher contacted my mother and emphasized that the camp experience was more than money. It was camaraderie. It was a date with Nature that an inner-city kid like me was missing. My mother was sold on the idea, and I was drafted.

But my chemistry teacher was right: I loved the experience. As it turned out, it also changed my life, several times over: when I chose a medical school and, later, when it came time to choose my specialty. This camp was blessed to have the best medical staff of any camp anywhere. Dr. Saul Krugman, the chairman of pediatrics at NYU School of Medicine, was also the camp's doctor after the Second World War. Academic physicians didn't earn much then; the only raise one could get was extra vacation time. One could use this time to earn additional money at whatever enterprise one could find, so Dr. Krugman enhanced his income by working at the camp. When he became chairman, he was no longer the camp doctor, but he recruited physicians from his department at NYU. Over the course of the six summers that I worked there, I met some of the academic giants of pediatrics, now out in the woods, relying only on their stethoscopes, eyes, ears, and hands for their clinical acumen. Dr. Krugman would come up each weekend with his wife, a former head counselor at the camp. Mrs. Krugman was a most congenial, talkative, and interesting individual. Dr. Krugman was a model of the laconic, contemplative soul;

he listened a lot but spoke little. Ultimately, he convinced me to choose NYU over the other medical schools that accepted me. All it took was a simple admonishment: "No one turns down NYU!"

It was Dr. Krugman who set my course in my fourth year of medical school. I was no longer working in the camp, but I had friends who were still there and wanted to visit them. Dr. Krugman was still the camp weekend warrior. I asked if he could provide me with a ride one summer weekend, and he graciously agreed. In the car, he asked which specialty I was going to choose. I admitted that I was torn between pediatrics and internal medicine. His subsequent monologue filled the entire ride (two and a half hours). He argued that there was nothing that internal medicine had to offer that pediatrics couldn't as well. Pediatrics was a study of development; medicine, a study of physical and mental attrition. Pediatrics was a plan to avoid disease; medicine was a discipline to try to undo, often unsuccessfully, the disease that should have been prevented. Medicine had cancer patients, but so did pediatrics. Medicine had infections, but pediatrics had a more diverse collection of infections. Pediatrics had a host of genetic anomalies that were often no longer seen by the internists. He argued that pediatrics was every bit as academic as internal medicine, possibly more so. I didn't get a word in during the trip, despite never having heard more than a sentence from Dr. Krugman at any of our previous meetings. His passion about pediatrics tilted the balance.

Pediatrics would be for me. I enjoyed playing with children. I could tolerate adolescents, still a bane of my existence. I liked my fellow pediatricians. I looked forward to the science to which Krugman alluded. My mind now at rest, I applied for internships in pediatrics and ultimately found myself staying on at NYU. Forty years after entering NYU Medical School, *je ne regrette rien.* As for my current responsibility as a pediatrician, I hope I can be as convincing to a puzzled medical student as Dr. Krugman was for me.

WHO'S RESPONSIBLE HERE?

Suzanne Dixon, MD, MPH

A BABY WAS DEAD—one I had touched and even attempted to treat—and it seemed that I would have to pay the price for this tragedy. I wasn't quite sure whether everyone would come after me with machetes, or simply denounce me and throw rocks to drive me away. Dire consequences seemed likely, in any case. I was terrified as we approached the site of the funeral.

I had been in western Kenya for only about a week as a fellow in Child Development, doing research on child care and parenting as part of a multidisciplinary team. Having completed my residency at a prestigious institution and now holding a similarly prestigious fellowship, I felt pretty confident of my skills. In addition to research activities, I was to provide medical care for the pregnant women and children of the study site, a market village of about 2,100 people. This meant running weekly clinics and doing home (hut) visits to newborns — very basic and very much needed in this area, as any other care was over ten miles away and, even then, extremely limited.

I did my first newborn visit, examining a full-term infant without apparent abnormalities. The pregnancy had been without complications, according to my predecessor's notes. I presented the new mom with a terry bath towel and a Fanta orange soda pop, the agreed-upon appropriate gift for the occasion. As I walked away that night, I glowed with excitement, enthusiasm, and optimism about my ability to contribute in several ways. The cool weather of the highlands and the lush green of the tea and coffee fields seemed idyllic, exotic. Dab-and-wattle huts with thatched roofs and dirt floors dotted steep hillsides surrounding a small market area and a two-room, whitewashed building that served as the project headquarters. Life was good.

The next morning as I drove up to our center, I was met by the newly delivered mom, carrying her infant in her arms. Opening the wrap, I could see a gray, mottled baby in extremis. Digging in my supplies, I found some chloramphenicol and penicillin, which I injected as fast as I could get them ready. I put the mom, baby, and a terrified research assistant in the car and drove like a maniac over mud-rutted roads to the district hospital. A nurse grabbed the infant, and after my explanation, the

Danish physician assured me they would do all they could. He agreed with my diagnosis, that neonatal sepsis (severe infection of the newborn) was the most likely explanation.

The following day, the mom and a bundle met me at the hospital entrance. The infant had died in the night, and she wanted a ride back to her home for the child's burial. When I dropped her off, she began that terrible keening that marks death in much of the world. Her voice was joined by those of other women. The hills caught the echo, and the noise was terrifying.

At the debriefing back at the village headquarters, I was assured by our anthropologist leader that I would not be blamed for the death and that I should attend the funeral with him the next day. Anthropologists love funerals, where so much is revealed about history, relationships, interactions, and gossip. I, on the other hand, hate funerals. As a health care provider, I was socialized to see death as a defeat, the enemy — and I don't like to look the enemy in the face. As a pediatrician, I expect most children to be well and stay well. I had also been socialized to take responsibility, to be in charge, and to anticipate and avoid catastrophe. So I was carrying a big burden of guilt as I walked to the hut where a large crowd was gathered for the funeral rituals and burial of the infant in front of the dwelling. Hence my fear of stoning, being sliced and diced, or even being boiled in a cauldron like a cartoon character.

All the distant relatives gathered, conversing in small

groups with the bereaved mother, secluded in her hut. A goat was roasting, and home-brewed beer was being shared all around in large, common bowls with reed straws. My senior colleague, Bob, was brimming with excitement at this anthropological opportunity and was taking notes furiously, an interpreter sitting between us. I couldn't focus on the translation of the proceedings, as I was waiting to be accused of killing the infant with my touch and my meager ministrations. Suddenly the talk got very animated and pretty scary. Someone pulled the pole on the top of the roof down, and there was a communal gasp at this action. The significance was beyond me in my terrified state. People were charging in and out of the yard, and a senior man appeared, as if to take charge. Apparently he had come a great distance to participate. Bob said, "Isn't this exciting?" All sorts of accusations were discussed: adultery by the mother, witchcraft by the grandmother, and theft by the father and his relatives. Malfeasance by the mother's cowives also was brought into it. The transgressions of two generations back were aired with vigor and great detail. Finally, a pause. Our interpreter said that all had agreed ("It is famous," is how he phrased it) that the infant's death was clearly caused by the mother's adultery and was entangled in all the sins of the past, involving the father and paternal grandfather and several brothers as well. No one mentioned me at all.

I walked away, relieved that I had not been hacked apart, as I'd imagined in my panic and guilt. The intensity of that moment taught me a lot about what is now known as the "subjective diagnosis" of the patient and family. The serious illness or death of a child is always painful and glaringly out of the proper order of things. That incomprehensible situation calls out for some explanation, when often there is no real explanation. Every family digs into themselves and back into history for something concrete to which to assign this inexplicable loss. Explanations of the pathophysiology of disease and recurrence risk numbers usually are hollow in these circumstances, in every family, everywhere.

Years later, I was doing an interview with a mom whose child had a complex genetic condition. I was with the third-year resident who had cared for this child since birth and knew the family well. Since the goal of this teaching session was to explore explanatory models of disease, the resident and I had discussed ahead of time how the family understood the child's condition with all its ramifications. He assured me that they had had several conversations about the cause, about genetic risk, and about the possibility of recurrence and that the mom would recite all that he and the other experts had imparted to her. Since she was an assistant professor at the university, he was quite confident that she had gotten things straight. In the interview, we talked with her about the complex care issues related to her needy child, the experts that she had consulted, all the changes this birth had demanded of her and her husband, and even the financial pressures they were experiencing. At a pause, I asked her what she thought had caused her child's condition. Without hesitating, she said it was because she had worn too-tight pantyhose in the early part of her pregnancy. I didn't challenge that, as I was afraid I'd have to resuscitate the resident, who literally lurched in his chair at that response.

At our debriefing, the resident admitted that he had never asked her what she thought had caused the condition. He had assumed that he was the one with the answers. I assured him that there is always guilt in the air when a child is ill or impaired. It's just a matter of finding out where it is attached and who is thought to be responsible.

I have had the privilege of taking my pediatric career to many parts of the world, in many different settings, and that has enriched my life immensely. Travel broadens, they say, and I endorse that big-time. So much is the same as families struggle to care for their kids under great burdens and against terrible odds. I watch as they instill the core of culture in their offspring — not just the exotic languages and strange rituals but the psychological structures, too. I'm there to facilitate that process, as well as to help keep children safe from disease and injury. And all families are partners in that process. We are all responsible.

Cuba

Lee Savio Beers, MD

CHICKENS WANDERING into the emergency room. Iguanas chasing down my fiancé. Land crabs crawling across my feet at the movies… This was not how I'd imagined beginning my career as a pediatrician.

During my senior year of college, while applying to medical schools, I made the decision to accept a scholarship with the U.S. Navy. Financially, it was an easy decision — tuition, books, supplies, and a monthly stipend to attend any medical school in the country in exchange for four years of military service as a physician. I also saw the scholarship as an opportunity to do something worthwhile with my training and give something back to the community. I liked the idea of using my skills to help children and families who had unique stresses and needs. No one in my immediate family had ever been in the military (and those who know me would agree that I certainly don't fit the stereotype of a no-nonsense, politically conservative naval officer), but I have always had great respect for the men and women in uniform who choose to serve our country.

I knew there was a chance I could be deployed overseas or somewhere remote. But like most 20-year-olds, I wasn't really looking that far ahead. Besides, I reasoned, I can do anything for four years. Considering my options, I decided that I would rather have four years living somewhere I didn't like than a lifetime of loan repayment. I have always been fairly flexible and assumed I would adjust and make the best of it. As it turns out, I had the opportunity to do just that.

I completed my pediatric training in a small program at a naval hospital in Virginia. During the winter of my last year of residency, while my civilian counterparts were busy scheduling job or fellowship interviews, my fellow residents and I were on the phone, pleading our cases with the Navy, where our superiors would decide where we would go next and what we would do. As you may imagine, there were places that were desirable to move to and places that most wanted to avoid at all costs. The naval hospital at Guantánamo Bay in Cuba was one of the latter. Even in the late 1990s, before "Gitmo" achieved its current level of infamy, it was not the top choice for many military pediatricians, and that year, it was the top choice for no one. My arguments against being assigned there were apparently the least compelling, and one afternoon while preparing for afternoon rounds, I got a page that my orders to Guantánamo Bay would be arriving soon. After a frantic call to my boyfriend, who was later to become my husband (after enduring many flights on Air Sunshine — where passengers were seated by weight in order to keep the plane balanced), and a weekend of moping, I began to prepare, mentally and physically, for 18 months at an isolated naval base.

Guantánamo Bay, even then, was a unique place. Located on the southeastern tip of Cuba, the base itself is completely isolated from the rest of the island, with barbed wire and armed guards surrounding its boundaries. The base sits in a valley, and it is very dry, not the lush tropical oasis you might imagine; the ground is covered with tumbleweed and cacti, and overall, it looks like a desert that happens to be surrounded by water. There are any number of animals roaming the base, including the aforementioned chickens, iguanas, and land crabs, as well as a very ugly rodent euphemistically called the "banana rat" (based on the fact that it looks like a gigantic rat, with feces the shape of small bananas). At the time, the base had about 3,000 residents, who were a mix of active duty personnel, civilian contractors, and family members.

There was one pediatrician for the base, and that was going to be me. Suddenly, knowing that I would be the first one called for any pediatric emergency, all of my experience in critical care seemed much more relevant. If a baby needed to be resuscitated or a toddler suffered serious trauma, I would be in charge — a daunting responsibility for someone who hadn't even taken her board exam yet. Additionally, many lab tests and radiologic studies (such as a CT scan or MRI) were not available at the hospital, and certainly no pediatric specialists were assigned to the base. Anyone needing these services would have to be flown back to the continental United States for treatment. As a physician, I would be very much on my own. I decided fairly quickly that if I had to be there, I was going to be as prepared as I could and make the best of it.

One of the first things I did after arriving on base (after going to my room to cry) was to take inventory of the inpatient ward and delivery room. I wanted to be sure that I had everything I needed in working order and that I knew where it all was. I chased down the nurse anesthetist to ask for a tutorial on the infant ventilator, which looked ancient and made me nervous. "It definitely works," he assured me. It was an old machine, so there were a few tricks to make sure you could control the pressure, but as long as you knew those it would be fine. He was in a bit of a hurry, as he himself was getting ready to transfer off the island, but he promised me he would be sure the new anesthesiologist knew all about it. Additionally, he told me, he had already placed an order for a new, top-of-the-line ventilator that could be used with neonates, and it should be arriving any time now. I wasn't sure I was comfortable with this situation, but since he was much more senior than I was, I took him at his word and hoped I never needed to actually use this old ventilator.

Months went by, and still the new ventilator did not arrive. Every time I asked about it, I was told that sometimes it took a really long time for supplies to get delivered to the base and that I shouldn't worry. Then, one afternoon, a pregnant visitor to the island went into preterm labor. While the obstetrician examined her in the emergency room, the anesthesiologist and I went to set up the old ventilator, just in case. Apparently, the machine required a few more "tricks" than I was initially led to believe, and the anesthesiologist had never gotten that promised briefing from his predecessor. After playing around with the elderly machine for a bit, he leaned down to peer at the settings while he turned it on. As soon as he flipped the on switch, a loud, forceful burst of air shot out, literally knocking his contact lens out of his eye and six feet across the room. Amazingly, there was no damage to the anesthesiologist's eye, but that was the end of that ventilator — just as we might actually need it. I had visions of hand "bagging" a preterm infant for eight hours while waiting for the medevac transport to arrive.

I learned a number of important lessons that day. First, if something is really important, don't ever take people at their word about it, no matter how trustworthy you think they are. At the risk of sounding melodramatic, your patient's life may depend on it. Always double-check the crucial things for yourself and make sure you know how everything works — there may not be anyone else available to help you when you need it, or the person who is there may not know either. Had I had spent more time playing with that ventilator myself, I would have realized that it was not functioning.

Second, don't be afraid to stand up for yourself or question authority. I may have been a brand-new pediatrician when I arrived in Guantánamo Bay, but I was the most experienced pediatric provider on base. From my first week there, I had been forced to stand up to senior military officers for what I thought was right for my patients, and I should have done it this time, too. If I had asked more questions, or insisted on confirming that a new ventilator had been ordered, we might not have been in this fix. Ultimately, I was responsible for the health of the children on the base, and I would have never forgiven myself if something bad had happened because I didn't want to seem pushy. I'd rather have had someone mad at me than not have had what I needed for my patients.

There were times later when I remembered this and didn't hesitate to insist on what I thought was the best treatment, even if someone else thought I was overreacting. I referred very few patients off the base for treatment, and was willing to discuss alternate options, but I learned to trust my medical judgment and I stood my ground. Since leaving the Navy, I have worked in a very underserved area of Washington, D.C.; many of my patients do not feel empowered to stand up for their own health, and the lessons I learned as a new pediatrician help me to be their advocate.

Third, if something goes wrong (which it inevitably will), take the time to reassess, use all your resources, and keep looking for a solution. Sometimes I remember this lesson in the moment, and sometimes I don't remember it until afterward when I think about what I could have done better. But I always remember it.

That day in the emergency room, after we located the anesthesiologist's contact lens, the team mobilized quickly to find a working neonatal ventilator. Because of our unusual geographic location, we couldn't just call the hospital up the road for a loaner or transfer the patient elsewhere. Instead, we identified a routine flight coming from another military base, which happened to have a Level III NICU. They were able to rush someone down to the airport with a spare ventilator for us to borrow until a new one could be ordered (since it turned out that the original order had never actually been placed). The good news was that the mother's contractions ultimately stopped and we never had to use the machine — but we would have been ready for that preterm baby if the labor hadn't stopped. And many months later, when an infant was born on base with severe hydracephaly, I was very glad that we had all of the equipment that we might need.

At the end of 18 months, I was overjoyed to be returning home. As I got on the ferry to the airport, I took one last look back and then looked out over the water for the rest of the trip. That year and a half had been long and filled with many difficult and depressing times. It is not a time I would ever choose to repeat, but it defined me as a pediatrician. Far away from specialists, and even many basic medical resources, I was forced to refine my diagnostic skills, trust my instincts, and learn from my mistakes. In a small, closely knit community, I had the opportunity to get to know my patients and their families at a much deeper level. They depended on me, and I learned a great deal from them. I was the sole provider of pediatric services on base, and I had to delve into many areas of training and administration — all of which have shaped the remainder of my career as an academic pediatrician. So I guess in the end, I was right. I made the best of it, and it made the best of me.

What Do You Tell the Aspiring Pediatrician?

Bryan Vartabedian, MD

I RECENTLY HOSTED a young premed student, Amy, in my office for a day. She was a recent graduate of the University of Texas and an aspiring pediatrician. I am a pediatric gastroenterologist, and a mutual friend thought I would be a good person for Amy to shadow and ask questions about a career in medicine.

I met Amy in my office one morning before going to the clinic. As we talked, I learned that she had been a literature major who came to consider medicine late in college, after losing her father to cancer. Amy was drawn to medicine after spending many months in and out of hospitals and clinics with her father. As an observer of doctor-patient relationships, she felt that she had a sense of what might make a compassionate physician.

We jumped right in at the clinic. We started with the simple step of having her see what I do on a daily basis. We saw patients together. I pointed out the unusual diseases that come to my pediatric gastroenterology practice, as well as the bread and butter pediatrics that makes up most of my day. I reflected a little bit on the complexity of the parent-child relationship. We saw a child with abdominal pain due to refractory Crohn's disease, as well as a child with abdominal pain due to the stress of divorcing parents. Within 15 minutes, we saw a child who went to the bathroom too often — and another who refused to go. Our morning showcased both the pleasures and the pressures of caring for children with chronic disease. And as the morning progressed, Amy was exposed to some clinical scenarios that were a bit more bizarre.

One of my chronic reflux patients appeared in the office for a routine follow-up appointment. Reviewing the history for Amy's benefit, I rattled off my laundry list of childhood heartburn questions, looking for signs of hidden trouble. And then I asked if there was anything else going on. As it turns out, there was. Colby had taken to pooping in the back yard. But Colby wasn't the family dog; he was my four-year-old patient. I could tell that the mom had been itching to drop this one on me since coming through the door. She mentioned it in a casual, matter-of-fact sort of way, as if she wasn't very concerned — but I got the feeling that this was the true reason for the visit...what doctors call the "hidden agenda." His reflux was stable and it was too early for a follow-up, so I had already been feeling a little suspicious. The mom looked at me, hoping that I'd assure her that this was just another speed bump on the road of parenthood. She was hoping for some sort of feel-good feature article in a parenting magazine, where no one does anything wrong and everything's just a phase.

Now, Colby was toilet trained in the traditional sense. It seems his deviancy began one day while watching the cows at his family's ranch. Colby took it upon himself to go *au natural.* The deal was sealed as Grandma and Grandpa looked on with amusement. But it became less amusing when this potty al fresco style evolved as his preferred mode of elimination, even after dark or during backyard barbecues.

I did my best to maintain an appearance of warm, empathetic concern, while at the same time imagining this kid squatting like a dog at the family picnic. I finally had to let my façade crack and admit, flat out, that this was one of the most bizarre things I had ever heard. And thus, I offered Amy her first pediatric clinical pearl: that when all else fails with a family, downshift into bald-faced honesty and you'll almost never go wrong.

So what did I tell Colby's mother? I reassured her that I felt his open-air preferences were nothing more than old-fashioned behavioral conditioning. I suggested that the next time her child engaged in bizarre, inappropriate behavior, it should not be reinforced with smiles and warm laughter.

I wondered if this case had been too much for Amy. But fortunately, the remainder of the morning brought more straightforward pediatric gastrointestinal cases.

This is how you showcase your life's work—you let someone follow and observe. Like a docent whose only obligation is to point out notable exhibits in passing, I found all of this relatively easy. But then came the moment when we broke for lunch. I knew it was here that the student would confront me with the tougher questions about life as a doctor. And so it happened: "Would you recommend medicine as a career, and are you happy?"

Sitting with Amy brought me back to my earlier years, contemplating life as a doctor. This lunch was a bit like my medical school interviews, when I was put under a dissecting microscope and quizzed about why I was choosing to become a physician. Like so many applicants, I wasn't precisely sure why I wanted to do what I was applying for, and my responses were contrived and rehearsed. Like Amy, all I knew for sure was that medicine seemed exciting and ripe with opportunity.

My start in medicine came inside the locked doors of a child psychiatric unit, as a nurse's aide. After four years of college and a wandering career itinerary, I found my way into the local psychiatric hospital on the 3-to-11 shift. The hospital was the Westwood Lodge, a private facility in the Boston suburbs. A friend had suggested that I might be good with the patients. He was right. My work there unearthed a capacity to connect with sick, stressed-out patients. The role of healer came fairly easily to me, even though it was limited at the time to one-on-one interactions with escalating, delusional patients. I thought medicine would be a good fit and subsequently found my way into medical school.

Looking back, I've always thought that my earliest work at the Westwood Lodge served me well in my career. After all, any pediatric gastroenterologist worth his salt will tell you that the problems of the psychiatric patient are just extreme manifestations of what every parent experiences from time to time when raising children. And how a pediatrician deals with the concerns and preoccupations of his patients' parents can define the patient's outcomes.

Now nearly 20 years later, I was forced to revisit the question of career choice — but this time with the advantage of retrospection. When I began my training in medicine, the crisis in malpractice was only beginning to brew, and pressures from insurance payers were just beginning to rise. The Internet didn't exist, and the opinion of an individual physician carried more clout than it does today. Physicians were able to maintain small businesses with returns that made the sweat and pressure of caring for the ill worth it in ways other than just feeling good.

Sitting with Amy, I found myself faced with a dilemma: How did I temper her idealistic fantasy with my own experiences and the realities of practicing today? How does a profession arguably in crisis recruit its next generation, when it's unclear what the future holds? When you're 22, it's hard to process the reality of what you may face at 44.

During our lunch, I tried to explain that, over the course of one's career, goals, interests, and motivations will change. The need for security and prestige will ultimately give way to a drive for happiness. The intense motivation to spend every waking moment focused on your training will give way to a desire for balance. The unusual childhood cancers and genetic cases that fascinate you as a young, single pediatrician-in-training will haunt you when the day comes to have your own children.

And looking back, I've recognized that having children changes everything about the most important part of treating children — treating parents. While it's always hard for the childless pediatrician to understand, children really do change everything. Children balance you as a pediatrician and a person. They afford unique insight into the complicated dynamic that invariably occurs when parents present their child to you for help. Our life experiences shape the relationships we share with our patients and their parents. And parenthood for pediatricians is a good thing.

Beyond the insight is the practical angle of credibility that comes when you tell a parent that you, too, have kids. I can't count the number of times that as a young pediatrician, I had to sheepishly confess my lack of parenting experience. I welcomed the birth of my first son — not only for the life-changing energy that he brought me but also for the fact that I could finally speak from experience. It's during the most trying times that parents feel reassured by someone who's been there…someone who has faced the frustration of a screaming baby. While I don't treat these problems any differently than I did before my children were born, parents now see me as an insider — someone who can speak from true experience. Parents trusted me when I was younger. Parents trust me *more* now that I've been through it. I said this to Amy, who politely took it all in without entirely understanding what I was telling her.

The day that had seemed like a minor imposition at first ended up making me think about where I was and where I had come from. How was I different than I used to be, and how had I evolved as a healer?

Despite all of the changes and stages that come with the evolution of a seasoned clinician, what remains at the core is the personal connection that comes when parents put their child into your care. Where you work, what you earn, what the trial attorneys do to you, and how society sees you may be very different 25 years from now — but this unique, intimate feeling will always remain. The best doctors are addicted to this intimacy.

JAZMINE

Christine Gleason, MD

Toward the end of my first year of pediatric residency, I was assigned for one month to the "Mac House" rotation. McDonald House was the OB/GYN department building, and one floor was devoted to delivering babies — approximately 4,000 of them each year. This was one of the busiest rotations of the residency. The pediatric resident attended all C-section deliveries and any full-term delivery in which a problem was anticipated (most of these involved meconium-stained amniotic fluid). We were also in charge of all the normal newborns in the nursery, particularly those who didn't have an assigned pediatrician, which was the case for most of the 20 to 30 babies in our public university hospital nursery. We did the initial newborn exams on those babies, followed their feeding progress, talked to their mothers about "well baby care" and "anticipatory guidance," and did their discharge exams.

The Mac House beeper was like a hot potato. We residents couldn't wait to pass it off to the next resident when our shift was over. It went off constantly, summoning the resident to attend deliveries (these were always STAT pages), discharge newborns (at all hours of the day or night), or see a baby that just didn't look right. You knew that if you were carrying the Mac House beeper, you'd be paged every ten minutes or so, on average.

One of the good things about Mac House was that you could pick up newborns for your own panel of "continuity" patients. When we started our residency training, we'd each been assigned to an attending-led clinic team (mine was the Orange Team). Once a week, we were allowed to leave our inpatient rotation and see patients in our continuity clinics for an afternoon. We usually saw about six patients during each session. They were scheduled just as in a regular pediatrician's office, although a pediatrician would generally see at least twice as many kids as we did. If you picked up a newborn for your clinic during your internship year, you then had a chance to follow that child for three years and really get to know the child and the family. By this time, I had about 30 kids on my "panel" of patients. I'd inherited most from one of last year's graduating residents. Only a handful of them were "mine," and even fewer were infants. These latter

I had picked up during my rotations in the emergency department, where I'd quickly discovered that parents who didn't have a pediatrician often used the emergency room whenever their child had an acute illness. We'd try to get these parents to come to our continuity clinics for follow-up of their child's illness, and some of them stayed with us after that for their well child care. Now, however, was my big chance to pick up some newborns.

I was finishing up my delivery room note on a big, healthy baby girl who'd had some fetal distress but had turned out fine, when the beeper went off again — this time for the nursery.

"This is Chris Gleason returning a page," I said to Rosie, the unit clerk who answered the nursery phone.

"One of the babies has a temp," Rosie said, "and the nurses want you to check her out."

I sighed. If the "temp" (fever) was real, not caused by overheating the baby, then I'd have to start a septic workup and transfer the baby to the neonatal unit for antibiotics. At night, the unit staff would do the workup, but during the day, because there was an intern assigned to the nursery (me), our colleagues in the neonatal unit expected us to get most of the workup done before transferring the baby. This would really slow down my morning routine — I had at least a dozen babies who needed discharge newborn physicals so they could go home with their mothers.

When I arrived back at the nursery, the nurses led me to a roly-poly black baby sucking on her fingers in a bassinet. She didn't look very sick, but when I looked

at her bedside chart, I saw that her latest temperature —
39° C — had been circled in red. It was an axillary temperature, taken with the thermometer held under her arm. If
she had been overheated (usually by overzealous parents
wrapping the baby in three or four layers of clothing and
blankets), then a rectal temperature would be normal or
at least significantly lower than the axillary temperature.

"Have you done a rectal temp?" I asked the head
nurse hopefully.

"Of course, Chris; you know we always check that
first," she said somewhat smugly. "And it was the same as
the axillary temp — 39° C."

So, no matter how good the baby looked, she would
need a full septic workup: blood, urine, and spinal fluid
cultures. Before I got started, I'd need to talk to her
mother, not only to let her know what was going on but
to get her permission to do a spinal tap (to get a sample
of spinal fluid) and a suprapubic bladder tap (to get a
clean, uncontaminated sample of urine). After I finished
the procedures, I'd need to start an IV for her antibiotics.
Then I'd have to call the chief resident to let him know an
admission was coming, write a transfer note, and, finally,
wheel the baby over to the neonatal unit myself. If everything went smoothly, I could get the whole job done in an
hour. If not, who knew?

The baby's mother's name — Alma King — was written on a card taped to the baby's bassinet, along with the
baby's sex, birth weight, and length. I noticed a blank
space by the notation "Pediatrician" and realized that this

might be a golden opportunity for me to pick up a newborn patient for my continuity clinic roster.

I asked Rosie, the nursery unit clerk, where I could find Alma King's room, and she directed me to a large, four-patient room at the end of the hall. I had to call out Ms. King's name to be sure I talked to the right mother. A large, sleepy-looking black woman answered softly, "That's me." And then she furrowed her brow and asked, "Is there anything wrong?"

I introduced myself as the doctor taking care of all the babies in the nursery, and then I told her that her two-day-old baby girl had developed a fever.

"But you'd never know there was anything wrong with her," I reassured her worried mom. "She's just lying there happily sucking on her fingers as if she didn't have a care in the world."

"Could I have just held her too long and gotten her all heated up?" Alma asked hopefully, just as I had asked the nurse about the rectal temp.

"Well, that's not very likely," I said, trying to explain the similarity between the baby's rectal and axillary temperatures. "And with newborn babies, you can never be too careful. They can't tell us if something hurts. So when they have a fever, we always assume it's an infection and begin treatment with antibiotics. If it turns out to be a false alarm, then we can just stop the antibiotics and send her home."

"So, how are you going to find out if she has an infection?" her mother asked me quietly, looking down at her bedclothes, which she was now wringing in her hands.

I then explained the procedures I would need to do to get clean samples of her baby's blood, urine, and spinal fluid. She winced visibly when I explained the suprabubic bladder tap I'd need to do to get the urine sample.

"Do you really have to do that one?" she asked. "I can understand the blood test and the spinal tap, but it just sounds awful to me — you sticking a needle right through her stomach into her bladder."

Inwardly, I had to agree with her. Suprapubic bladder aspiration was one of the most barbaric neonatal procedures we ever had to do. But, as I explained to Ms. King, it was necessary if we wanted to get a clean sample, uncontaminated by organisms that normally existed on the skin or around the baby's tiny urethra.

"If we just tried to 'catch' a clean sample in her diaper or got a sample by putting a catheter into her bladder through her urethra, it would be really hard to interpret if the culture came back positive," I told her. "We'd wonder if she had a real bladder infection, which would mean ten days of IV antibiotics, or if we'd just gotten a contaminated specimen."

She said she wanted to know all the risks involved with the procedure before she'd agree to let me do it. I realized that I'd seriously underestimated this woman when I walked into the room. Normally, parents would simply accept what we told them and ask where they should sign, but this baby's mother wanted to know more. I pulled over a chair and spent the next 15 minutes trying to convince her that the procedure was really safe (and that yes, I'd done it myself at least a dozen times without any mishaps). In the end, though, she refused to give me her consent. She told me she was willing to accept the consequences; that is, her baby might have to stay in the hospital for ten days of IV antibiotics just because a questionable urine specimen turned positive.

I was impressed with this woman, but I was also annoyed and impatient. I'd spent a total of 30 precious minutes of my time talking to her, and to some extent, it was all for naught. And now I was far behind on my to-do list for the day. I gathered up the signed consent form for the LP and the unsigned one for the suprapubic bladder tap, and I headed for the door. She called after me.

"Take good care of my baby, Dr. Gleason. Her name's Jazmine, and she's all I've got in the world."

I promised her I'd do my best and assured her that I'd tell her the initial results, which I expected back by the end of the day. The culture results would take at least 48 hours, and the baby would be in the neonatal unit when they came back. By then, her mother would be discharged, and the staff in the neonatal unit would be the ones to discuss those results and the treatment plan with her. Most likely, I'd never see her again. So much for picking up newborns for my clinic panel.

It didn't take me long to get the blood work done, to do the spinal tap on little Jazmine, and to start her IV. I wrote a brief note and her initial antibiotic orders and then called the chief resident and told him I needed to send a baby over to the neonatal unit.

"Another hot one?" he asked.

"Well, as a matter of fact, yes. Maybe we need to check the thermostat in the nursery. This baby's totally fine. I'd be surprised if anything grew."

"So we have blood, urine, and CSF to check, right?" he asked.

"Well, sort of," I said. And I told him what had happened with the suprapubic bladder tap.

"The mom knows what's at stake here, right?" he said. "I mean, if there's a positive cath culture, we're going to have to treat the kid even if it's likely to be a contaminant. And then we'll have to work up the baby's kidneys and urinary tract, too—before she goes home."

I explained that she knew all that and she didn't care. She just didn't want me to stick a needle into her baby's bladder, and that was that.

So I wrote the transfer orders and wheeled the baby over to the neonatal unit, giving a brief verbal report to the intern who was admitting her. Once that was all done, I walked back to the nursery and plunged into my long list of discharge physicals and parent teaching sessions (which were very brief: bring the baby in if he/she is hot, yellow, or stops eating). At 4:00 PM, I crossed the last name off my list and sank into a chair in the resident charting area to finish up some paperwork.

My paperwork was interrupted by two delivery room calls, so I didn't finish it until 6:30. I was off that night and couldn't wait to get home, take a long, hot shower, and pour myself a glass of wine. On my way to the hospital parking lot, I was considering having cheese and crackers for dinner so I wouldn't have to stop at the grocery store when I suddenly remembered that I'd promised Jazmine's mother that I'd tell her the initial test results. I was anxious to get home, and I told myself that the intern from the neonatal unit had probably already talked to her and a visit from me would be a waste of time. But I'd promised her. I knew I'd have to go back to the hospital, call for the results, and then go talk to Alma King.

I decided to go to the neonatal unit first instead of the nursery. I was hoping that the intern had gotten all the results and written them in the baby's chart, which would save me the hassle of having to track them down. I lucked out. Everything was right there in the baby's chart when I located it at the nurse's station. The white blood cell count looked fine, and so did the spinal fluid. But the urinalysis had a few white cells and some blood and protein in it—not as many as you'd expect to see with a bladder infection but, still, a bit suspicious. I walked by Jazmine's room on my way over to the nursery and saw her mother standing by the baby's little crib, talking to Janet, the intern on call. As I walked over to the bedside, I was startled to see Alma point to me and explain to the intern, "There's Jazmine's doctor, Dr. Gleason. She took good care of my baby in the nursery."

I felt a little burst of pride. She actually considered me her baby's doctor. Then I realized that maybe it was because the little pink card taped to the crib, which had the baby's name, weight, and birth date on it, now had my name listed on the previously blank "Pediatrician" line. Oh well, I thought, it doesn't matter how she decided that I was Jazmine's doctor. I was just glad that she had, because now I had a chance to add a new baby to my continuity clinic panel, beating out the admitting intern on the unit.

I listened for a few minutes as Janet finished her explanation of the suspicious urine test results and answered Alma's questions. Then I told both of them that I would check on the culture results the next day and we could discuss the plans for Jazmine. Of course, that would really be the job of the daytime intern, but I wanted to do what a real pediatrician would do. I left the unit feeling that I'd made the right decision to return to the hospital, in more ways than one.

The next day I couldn't wait to check Jazmine's test results and was thrilled when I saw that all the cultures were negative (or "no growth") so far. But my elation was short-lived; Jazmine's intern in the neonatal unit called me the following day to say that her urine culture had turned positive. Everyone suspected that there was a contaminant, both because it had been a "cath" specimen and because true positive cultures usually turned positive within 24 hours. But we all knew that we'd have to assume that it was real and that Jazmine would need IV antibiotics for another eight days. I reminded her mother that we usually did a couple of tests when babies finished antibiotics for bladder infections — just to make sure that they didn't have a kidney or bladder defect, which would make it more likely for them to get another bladder infection.

For the next week, I checked in on Jazmine and her mother every day, usually after I'd finished my work at Mac House. Alma had been discharged the day after Jazmine had been admitted to the neonatal unit and she essentially moved into Jazmine's room, sleeping on a foldout chair by her baby's crib. Jazmine continued to thrive, nursing well and going through only two IVs during her entire antibiotic course (a significant challenge, with a newborn's tiny veins). As the last day of her antibiotics drew near, the team in the neonatal unit asked my opinion about doing those tests we usually did before babies went home. It was the first time I was ever "consulted" on one of my patients, and I felt a real thrill. I read as much as I could about neonatal urinary tract infections and bladder or kidney defects and came to the conclusion that since Jazmine's infection wasn't likely to be real, the yield of these tests would likely be very low and we could forgo them.

I sat down with Alma to discuss my conclusions with her. I'd gotten to know her quite a bit better during Jazmine's hospitalization. She'd gradually shared a few details of her life with me, including the fact that the baby's father was in jail and she was on welfare but working on her high school equivalency diploma so that she could get a job and give Jazmine a better life than she'd had. She listened carefully as I explained why we usually did a renal ultrasound and a voiding cystourethrogram in babies who'd had a urinary tract infection. And she listened even more carefully as I explained why I didn't think we needed to do these tests on Jazmine.

"I trust you to make the best decision for my baby," she said, looking me straight in the eye. "That's why I chose you to be her doctor."

Suddenly, my clinical judgment, based upon the "evidence" I'd gleaned from the medical literature, seemed pretty arbitrary. Did I trust my own judgment as much as she did? And then I asked myself a question that I've continued to ask in similar moments of professional self-doubt over the years: What would I do if this were *my* baby? And I felt very comfortable with my decision. I told the team on the neonatal unit that I didn't think we needed to do those tests, and that I'd discussed the plan with the baby's mother and she'd agreed. Jazmine would be discharged without any prophylactic antibiotics and without the follow-up kidney tests — primarily because we all thought that the positive urine culture she'd had was most likely a false positive result. I would see the baby two weeks after discharge in my continuity clinic.

And so Jazmine became the first newborn in my continuity clinic. By the time I was a third-year resident, I'd have accumulated over two dozen newborns during my hospital rotations, but Jazmine was my first and, as it turned out, my most memorable. When I saw her at the two-week checkup I'd arranged, I couldn't believe how big she'd gotten — a pound heavier than her birth weight already. I told Alma what a great job she was doing and answered her questions about things such as diaper rash and nighttime crying jags.

Alma brought the baby faithfully to all the scheduled

well child checks, and I carefully administered all the scheduled baby shots and blood tests. Jazmine got sick only once — with an ear infection when she was a year old. I'd picked up the reddened eardrum on her routine 12-month checkup, and Alma was relieved that I'd found an explanation for Jazmine's increased fussiness and pulling on her right ear. The rest of her physical was fine, at least according to the brief notes made in her clinic record — something I was to pore over later on.

Three months later, I saw Jazmine again for her scheduled 15-month checkup. This was usually a pretty short visit, and the main event was the first MMR vaccine (measles, mumps, and rubella). I had a very busy schedule in the clinic that day, and Jazmine was the last patient on my list. It was close to 5:00 PM — closing time — when I walked into the exam room and sat down across from Alma, who was holding Jazmine in her lap. In answer to my standard 15-month checkup questions, she told me that Jazmine had taken her first steps just a month ago and could now walk across the room without holding onto anything. She could say several words, including "mama," "hi," and "NO," and she was a picky eater — except when it came to ice cream. I reviewed her growth, which was excellent, and then went over the usual 15-month "anticipatory guidance" topics with Alma, such as making sure all harmful household substances were out of Jazmine's reach, including boiling pots of water on the stove. I briefly examined Jazmine while she was in Alma's lap — I found that toddlers did much better with that approach than with trying to lay them down and hold them still on the examining table. I couldn't get a very good abdominal exam. Jazmine wasn't about to hold still, plus she was pretty ticklish. I told Alma that I'd done the important things on the exam and that Jazmine had passed with flying colors. I'd postpone a thorough abdominal exam until her 18-month visit, when she might be a bit more cooperative.

As I got the syringe and vial out to give Jazmine her MMR shot, Alma said, "I nearly forgot to tell you, Dr. Gleason; she has a sore spot on the front of her thigh. I don't remember her hurting herself there and there's no bruise, but if I press on the spot, she says 'ow' and pulls her leg away. You reminded me of it when you got out the shot stuff, because you usually give her the shot in her leg."

I held Jazmine's chubby little leg in my lap and pressed on the spot Alma had indicated. Jazmine jerked her leg away and started to cry. I was perplexed. There was no irregularity of the bone, no swelling or bruise over that spot, and no sign of an injury above or below it, either. I asked Alma to bring Jazmine out into the hall and put her down so I could see her walk. My clinic preceptor, Dr. Mack, happened to walk by as Alma put Jazmine down and walked a few feet away. Jazmine immediately toddled over to Alma's open arms — no problems at all.

"What's up, Chris?" Dr. Mack asked, looking at his watch. It was closing time, and I had to get over to the emergency department to begin my overnight shift. I told him what Alma had told me — which I'd confirmed myself. I also told him that I hadn't found anything wrong, although I remembered suddenly that I hadn't really done a complete exam, thinking of her abdomen. He reached down and scooped up Jazmine in his arms, playing with her for a minute so she'd relax. Then, he too pressed on the spot that Alma pointed out to him, and Jazmine once again pulled her leg away and started to cry.

"She needs an X-ray," Dr. Mack said, "just to be on the safe side."

I felt my insides turn suddenly cold. Could this be a sign of something bad? And had I missed it?

I rushed to the charting room to get an X-ray requisition and hurriedly filled it out.

"X-ray right leg; point tenderness over right anterior femur. Rule out bone lesion."

Dr. Mack knew I had to get to the ED. He said he'd take Alma and Jazmine over to radiology for the X-ray and promised he'd phone me with the results.

"What about her shot?" Alma asked, and I saw that she now directed her question at Dr. Mack, who had explained the need for the leg X-ray while I was filling out the requisition. He had such a wonderful bedside manner, and he'd clearly assumed the care of my patient. He was my preceptor, and of course this was the way it should be, but I suddenly felt very "junior" and inexperienced. It seemed pretty apparent to me, and I think to Alma, too, that now that the situation had gotten serious, a "real" doctor was needed.

"If everything's fine on the X-ray," Dr. Mack explained, "then I'll give her the shot before you go home." Alma didn't ask what would happen if everything was not fine on the X-ray.

I said good-bye to Alma and Jazmine; Alma just waved distractedly at me and gazed anxiously at Jazmine's leg. I hurried over to the ED and plunged quickly into the stack of waiting patients — mostly kids with minor injuries and illnesses. I cleaned out lots of earwax on my ED shifts so that I could get a better look at the kids' eardrums. About two hours later, I got a page, and when I called the number displayed on my beeper, Dr. Mack answered the phone. I braced for the worst, and I got it.

"She has a lytic bone lesion, Chris."

I felt as though the breath had just been sucked out of me.

"Where do you think the primary is?" I asked, referring to the metastatic tumor she must have. I tried not to let my emotions spill over into my voice, but tears were welling up in my eyes and I swallowed hard. Dr. Mack said that neuroblastoma was the most likely diagnosis; when it spread, it often went to the bone. Neuroblastoma is a tumor of the adrenal glands, which sit right above each kidney. I suddenly flashed back 15 months, to Jazmine's first hospitalization. Could this cancer have been there when she was born? And, I thought irrationally, could we have seen it if we'd done that renal ultrasound — the test I'd recommended *not* doing because I thought it was so unlikely that she'd had a bladder infection? It was an irrational thought, because I knew that although neuroblastoma could be diagnosed in newborns, it is usually considered because the baby had characteristic skin lesions — which Jazmine never had — and is usually benign or at least eminently treatable. Unlike neuroblastoma in a toddler that had already spread to the bone, which was usually fatal.

Jazmine would be admitted that night to the toddler unit so that all the necessary tests could be done and treatment could be started — usually beginning with surgery and staging of the tumor. As Dr. Mack went on, it was so clear to me that he was in charge, which was as it should be — he was my clinic preceptor and ultimately responsible for all my clinic patients. I told him that I would stop by her room in the morning, after my ED shift was over. Dr. Mack said he was sure that Alma would appreciate that.

I did stop by Jazmine's room the next morning, carrying an extra Styrofoam cup of coffee in case Alma hadn't had a chance to get down to the cafeteria. Jazmine wasn't there. She was already in the operating room, having a thorough physical exam (no one else had been able to palpate her abdomen either) and various painful tests done — all under anesthesia.

Alma sat in the chair by her crib, looking exhausted and dazed. She accepted the cup of coffee but didn't take a sip. She just held the warm cup in her hands and breathed in the steam.

"Do you think it was there when she was born?" she

whispered, with despair in her voice. So she'd been think-ing about that, too.

I confessed that I'd had the same thought, but I told her what I knew to be true: that neuroblastoma in the newborn just doesn't present that way.

"That's what Dr. Mack told me," she said, "but I just wanted to ask you because you were there back then. You were her very first doctor."

The only word I really heard was *were*. We both knew I wasn't going to be her doctor anymore, and I felt a deep sense of loss.

"She was my very first newborn continuity patient," I told Alma then.

"I knew that," Alma said. "The nurses in the nursery explained how we could pick one of you training doc-tors to be our baby's doctor if we wanted. I picked you because you had such a nice face, and you spent so much time with me, explaining about Jazmine's fever and every-thing. And I wish you could still be her doctor — her can-cer doctor."

I assured her that I would still be her doctor — for her well child care once she became well again. And of course, I told her that I would visit whenever Jazmine was in the hospital. In those days, most pediatric cancer care took place in the hospital, not in the outpatient setting, as it does today. I knew I would have lots of chances to visit Jazmine and her mother.

Alma put down her coffee cup and reached out to grasp both of my hands in hers.

"Pray for my baby, Dr. Gleason," she pleaded. "Pray for her hard."

Jazmine died six months later in the pediatric ICU, held tightly in her mother's arms.

FORSAN

Dipesh Navsaria, MD, MPH, MSLIS

Forsan et haec olim meminisse juvabit.
(Perhaps someday you will rejoice to recall even this.)
—Virgil, *The Aeneid*, Book I

IT WAS 8:00 ON A December morning, just a couple of days before Christmas. My last prevacation call night in the newborn intensive care unit was drawing to a close. This particular night had been worrisome. I had two very small preemies side-by-side in one corner of the unit, both, oddly enough, with the same first name. One, J.R., had been my patient since I had come on service and was still very tenuously alive and struggling to gain weight in the face not only of her prematurity, but also a patent ductus arteriosus (PDA), an opening between the pulmonary artery and the aortic arch, a remnant of fetal circulation that refused to close despite medication.

J.D., the other baby, had a similar story and occupied the bed spot next to J.R. She wasn't one of "ours" but was a transfer from another hospital who had come to us with the same open ductus, also persisting in the face of several rounds of medication. The plan had been for them both to have their PDAs ligated, or tied off surgically on the same day, while the surgeon, staff, and equipment were all available. This had happened the previous morning, and both had done well through their early postoperative courses.

I checked on them both multiple times through the night and was reassured — mostly. J.R. was doing okay, but J.D. had some oddly low blood pressures at times, though then they would come back up on their own. The nurse and I agonized over her on an hourly basis and promised each other to keep a close watch. The neonatologist had stayed in-house that night, and he had come by to check on both babies several times as well. We looked them over, discussed the numbers, and opted to continue to watch, albeit a bit nervously. I was glad he was there, because it wasn't a clear-cut situation — in cases such as this, years of experience and judgment are important.

As the dawn approached, a sense of relief spread over me. The long night was over, and after postcall morning rounds, I would be able to go home and enjoy a well-deserved few days off in the midst of my busy intern year. I started going from patient to patient, getting my numbers together, double-checking my calculations in the postcall haze. I was checking labs on the computer in the resident work area when, suddenly, everything went bad.

The neonatology fellow came striding out and declared that J.D. was "one sick little kid." He showed me the printout from the routine morning blood gas that had just been drawn. While I'm sure there have been lower pH values in the NICU before, this was the lowest I'd ever seen. There are many reasons for a low pH, but in essence, the blood becoming this acidic is a sign that something is profoundly wrong — this was the cry of millions of stressed cells struggling against some great duress. What was particularly remarkable was that there was no change in her vitals or clinical exam at this point.

What followed felt like a massive blur — in some ways, it lasted only a few minutes; in others, it was endless. It was not long before J.D.'s clinical status started to deteriorate. She went into cardiac arrest. The neonatologist who had come on service that morning called a code, and around the baby's tiny, less-than-three-pound body we had about nine people. By some stroke of luck, we had the NICU pharmacist on hand, and a pediatric cardiologist who was doing an echocardiogram on another patient rolled the machine over and gave us an intra-code look at her cardiac function.

Despite the blur, I remember the looks on people's faces. I saw J.R.'s parents, huddled by their own baby's incubator, trying their best not to look at us but fully, acutely, and terribly aware that a life-and-death drama was going on — with a child who'd just had the same procedure as their little girl.

I was grateful that J.D.'s parents had come in just before she began to deteriorate. I told them about the blood gas then, but I don't think they entirely processed how serious this was. I recall them standing back as we started chest compressions. I myself could barely tell what was going on with the code as the neonatologist called out orders, but I did my best to keep them updated as they watched us.

There was a giddy moment when we brought back the baby's heart and restored a normal rhythm. A small cheer went up, although there was always the unspoken question: How long had her little brain been without sufficient oxygen? Granted, neonates are incredible, and their physiology can bounce back from situations that would have long ago killed you or me, but there are limits.

This, however, was not to be. Within a few minutes, she decompensated again, and we were back to manually ventilating her lungs and compressing her chest. We had been working on her for almost three hours when I saw the attending's face contort and her voice crack as she raised the possibility that it was time to stop. I knew this point had been coming for a long time, but I hadn't quite believed it until now, and I felt a lump form in my throat. The attending went over to talk to the parents and reviewed the situation, then raised that final, awful question that no parent should ever have to hear.

Their answer was that we should stop. I knew — we

all knew—that this was the right thing at this point. I've never been one to endorse fighting on in the face of overwhelming odds. But for a patient that was doing reasonably well...how awful! I thought about how they had brought their child to our hospital after getting her through those tenuous early weeks, and how they would be leaving without her. I can't possibly imagine exactly how they felt, but I'd like to believe that I tried my best to attend to their needs during the code, and I had spent much of the night watching over their daughter.

We cleared away the excess lines and medical equipment and prepared to move the baby so we could let the parents hold her as she slipped away. Once she was clear of her attachments to the medical world, I started to lift her, ready to turn and give her to her grieving parents. I found myself being stopped by one of the senior nurses, who had J.D.'s nurse step in and lift her, saying to me, "She's his nurse."

The mixed feelings of sadness, anger, and bewilderment washed over me. Yes, that was true, but why did that matter? I had been there at that point for 29½ long hours, and I felt I had some clear right to participate in the last moments of this child. Perhaps I was being selfish, or petty, but the message I got was that because I was a physician, I didn't have the authority to care.

This might not surprise those who are used to medical environments where there is an antagonistic relationship between nursing and medical staff. However, it did me—I generally got along with the NICU nurses very well, and there was seldom cause for disagreement or bickering. I didn't expect to be booted out of this process quite like this. My own hope to join in the parents' grieving for just a moment was kicked to the curb.

I stepped back, yielding to a group of four nurses who surrounded J.D.'s mother, arranging blankets and pillows. Helpless and with no one around me, I turned to the wall and began sobbing into my arm. After a few moments, I exited the NICU to the privacy of the resident call room and wept.

I was not as alone as I might have thought—bless their hearts, my two senior resident colleagues who had come in that morning and assisted with the code saw me leaving in tears and came to check on me. One of them, upon realizing that these were the last hours before I started vacation, took my notes from me and told me to go home. After 30 hours and the emotional exhaustion of watching a patient I'd agonized over die, I did so—after some brief, feeble words of protest, of course.

TO THIS DAY, I'm grateful for their clearheaded words and compassion. Why? Because, as deeply as this death affected me, no one else ever said anything that acknowledged my pain or the stake that I had in this patient.

While I'd had patients die before, as a student, my connection to them didn't happen to be particularly close. One patient of mine died when I was a physician assistant—but well, it all happened in another hospital, away from me, and I wasn't even involved in treating the illness that led to her demise. Residency, however, brings a great and terrible intensity to everything. The sheer crush of time spent in any one particular setting magnifies both the joy and despair of caring for patients.

A week later, when I returned to work, I was chatting with a couple of the nurses when one of them referred to J.D.'s death and began to tell me about it. The other nurse broke in, reminding her that I had been there, not just in the morning but through the whole night. Was I that invisible?

A few months later, while discussing another case with the attending who had been there in the morning, I had to remind her that I had been there for the entire thing. Was I so interchangeable that my presence there as a person meant nothing?

Medical education has slowly evolved over time, and the old-time dichotomy between medicine and nursing has blurred in both directions. And while the task of being a resident often means having lesser "stakes" in a patient than when you're an attending, there is certainly emotional investment in our patients. I'd like to believe that I'm a caring, involved physician. I'd like to hope that I do the right things. But to be locked out by old assumptions and lines in the sand — well, a small part of me died with that little girl that morning.

SOME REDEMPTION DID COME, in a sense, almost two years later. As the resident covering the regular nursery, I had just come on duty for the overnight shift. I walked into another drama, again of the type that only the NICU can generate. A child who had been born two days earlier had suffered a period of hypoxia and was clearly brain-dead, as verified by an EEG. The family, after long deliberation, had made the choice to withdraw life-sustaining care, although they were waiting for one more family member, who had been delayed by bad weather, to arrive from out of town. The baby, M, forced the issue by dislodging her endotracheal tube. The attending asked the family whether they wanted us to reintubate or to withdraw care at this point.

Once again, I remember their faces. The baby's mother contorted in tears, sobbing, saying that she couldn't go through this again. The baby's father, taciturn but also in pain, made the final statement that we should withdraw care. Again, just as two years prior, we began to remove lines and prepare to give a child to her parents for her final time with them.

I had just walked in on this situation, and I had little to no emotional connection with this patient. The other resident (who was actually assigned to the NICU) was a cross-cover and didn't know this family either. So, to some extent, I readied myself for being pushed out of the situation. I even stepped back to let the baby's nurse give her to her parents. They were allowed to take her to the family room, where they could sit, hold her, and spend their last moments together. I wandered away, my presence clearly unneeded at this point.

It was, however, not 15 minutes later that her nurse came and found me.

"The family thinks she's gone."

I quickly looked around, but the neonatologist and the NICU resident were nowhere nearby, probably attending to other pressing matters. I didn't want to do something that was technically the job of the NICU resident, but at the same time, I didn't want to leave this family waiting in the great pause between the moments that their child was living and dead.

I took a deep breath and asked the nurse to grab a neonatal stethoscope, and we walked to the room together. I rehearsed in my head precisely what I needed to do and say — this family would always remember this moment and the words that came out of my mouth. We walked in, and I briefly said hello, getting nods and looks of concern; my reason for being there required no announcement. I uncovered the baby's small, untimely stilled chest and listened for a while, the silence filling my ears. I looked at the clock and simply, quietly pronounced her dead for the first time in my career.

The parents exhaled as if they'd been holding their breath, and relief filled their faces. I sat with them for a moment, holding their hands and offering my condolences. The room was not filled with grief and agony as it had been at the moment they decided to withdraw care but rather with a small, quiet sense of stillness and release. We walked out, and later her nurse found me and thanked me for how I had handled things.

I don't know why this was different. Certainly there were obvious contrasts; M's parents had expected her to die, while J.D. had taken a sudden, unexpected turn for the worse. A planned, compassionate withdrawal of support is a very different ending from a code situation, with its feelings of failure and defeat. And, of course, the personalities of the people involved change and mesh in different ways. Or maybe there was some difference in me over those two years, some evolution. I don't know for sure.

Not for a second do I believe that these losses are truly mine; the tragedies belong to the grieving families, but there is undoubtedly a connection left asunder between provider and patient. The cold, objective perspective we learn in medical school doesn't always hold true — we contain human feelings: ego, love, compassion, and grief. In the act of bearing witness to others' loss, I can salute and honor that which once was and that which now is.

I do know, however, that after every death I hear about, I go out of my way to find my fellow residents and interns (as well as medical students), make sure they're okay, and let them know that if they need to talk, I'm here.

THE CARE OF STRANGERS

Rachel H. Kowalsky, MD

A BROTHER AND SISTER have run away from home — or
at least, they wandered away from their grandmother
in the Bronx and took the subway 17 stops, exiting at South
Street Seaport. They were found climbing over a railing to
get a better look at the boats. The brother, Rafael, hands
thrust deep into his pockets, is seven. His sister, Laura,
is four. She wears a raggedy sundress and pink sequined
shoes. Oblivious to the quorum of cops and case workers
their presence has summoned, they were ogling the fish
in the seaport's fish tank.

Their grandmother arrives in the emergency department. She is thin, anxious. She wears thick glasses and thick
heels. I break the news to her — we've had to call ACS, the

Administration for Children's Services, to investigate the family. Even if the children didn't run away — even if they only wandered off — they were improperly supervised.

The woman is indignant, frowning at me over her glasses. "We are *buena gente* — good people. You don't know anything about us!"

She's right; I don't know them. In my job as a pediatric emergency physician, I care for thousands of children and families in a year, entering their lives at critical moments and exiting just as quickly. While many patients develop a relationship with their doctor over months and years, a typical ER shift is between 8 and 12 hours — about as long as it takes to fly cross-country, charge a battery, or marinate a chicken. It takes longer for paint to dry on the hospital walls.

The grandmother is interviewed by the ACS social worker. The office door is closed, but I can still hear the escalating emotion from down the hall. Through the shouting and crying, I catch that phrase again: *buena gente*. When she emerges, the grandmother is crying. Laura, the four-year-old, pulls herself away from the fish tank, rushes over, drapes her arms around the old woman's neck, and then starts to cry herself. The woman and child add their tears to the general din of the ER. The medical student I am working with looks at me, distraught. "Maybe we shouldn't have called ACS."

I have a set of rules for taking care of strangers, and I lecture the student about Rule Number One: *Treat every family the same*. In this frenetic setting, I will never learn whether a family is *buena gente* or not, so I have to do the same thing for every little wanderer: call ACS. If the children had strayed from a picnic on the well-heeled Upper East Side, I'd have to do the same (and I have).

Then, because I have a few moments (and the medical student is a captive audience), I share Rule Number Two: *Learn one thing from each patient.* Rafael, the seven-year-old, has a benign heart murmur. I tell her to go and listen to it. That way, when she hears an abnormal murmur, she will know the difference. "See?" I expound. "You'll never see Rafael again, but he will influence your practice for years to come."

Rules one and two are basic. Anyone who went to medical school in the last century has been lectured on both of these topics. The more difficult task, when caring for strangers, is to inject humanity into these brief encounters — to pop in and out of people's lives with grace. Thirty minutes later, when my shift ends, I make an attempt. The children and their grandmother are sitting miserably in an alcove, situated directly between me and the door. "Good-bye," I say, standing uncertainly before them. Nobody looks up. I kneel down to Laura's eye level and offer her a sticker. She scowls at me. I accept my defeat.

The other rule of caring for strangers is one I learned as a resident in pediatrics. It was routine to cross-cover patients, or to care for a patient briefly, usually overnight or on a weekend. On weekdays, each patient had a primary resident, a resident who knew the patient well and was responsible for his or her care. But, despite being called "resident," no doctor truly lives in the hospital — and when the primary doctor went home, somebody had to assume care of those patients. This is true in essentially every hospital in the country, and it's why the cross-cover role exists. Cross-cover doctors, like ER doctors, must take care of children they do not know.

When I was a resident, we had systems in place to make cross-coverage as seamless as possible. For example, each patient had a weekly log with a column for each day of the week. Each day we recorded the vital signs and lab results, the child's medications and diet specifications, and any important events that had occurred. When we "signed out" a patient to the cross-cover, we handed that doctor the log. It became all-important — the patient's whole illness distilled into a few lines of text.

Despite all the organization, cross-coverage was always a delicate situation. Entering a child's hospital course *in medias res* felt like opening a novel to a random page or entering a movie theater halfway through the film. I learned to ask a lot of questions at sign-out so that I would never walk into a patient's room unprepared. And I became used to hearing "You don't know my son," or "You don't know what works for my daughter." Experienced parents would even say, as I came by to introduce myself, "I know — you're just cross-covering."

And then, a resident's nightmare: I was cross-covering Amanda Lopez the night she died. Amanda (not her real name) had a rare and virulent form of childhood leukemia. She was DNR (Do Not Resuscitate) and ALOC (Altered Level of Care). The latter meant that we were not to do anything invasive or painful, such as draw blood or put in IVs. She was to receive comfort measures only.

Boyd, my coresident, signed her out to me. Amanda's primary, Sam, was postcall—he had worked overnight the night before, going home at 11:00. So Boyd had covered Amanda. And now she was mine: double cross-coverage. She had been febrile all day, lapsing in and out of consciousness, her blood pressure falling. Boyd told me she was going to die. In fact, he had actually started the necessary paperwork for me: the death certificate, the organ donation papers, and the event note on the computer—the "event" being death. This is how it read: "Amanda is a 6-year-old female with leukemia. Status: post multiple rounds of chemotherapy, now with end-stage disease and presumed sepsis, on ALOC." I could write the rest later.

Amanda liked to wear ponchos. Her favorite was a nubby cream-colored poncho with navy stripes; it was way too big for her tiny body. I knew her but not well, the way I knew the kids in my apartment building. She had been in the hospital a long time. Her log had weeks and weeks worth of papers stapled together, but since she'd become ALOC, not much was written there. She had hollow cheeks, large, lovely eyes, and a wise, pointed chin. She was very close with her oncologist and with Sam, her primary—but neither of them was there. I was there.

I introduced myself to Amanda's parents. I said I was their doctor for the night. I asked whether Amanda was comfortable and if they needed anything. Amanda's mom asked whether Sam, her primary resident, was around. I said no. He was actually at a wedding, but I couldn't bring myself to say this. She nodded. I suppose on the scale of disappointments, this final one was small. She asked me for a glass of water for Amanda. *Ice?* I asked. *No thanks.* I stood around for a bit, watching her offer the water to Amanda. I remember that the girl's lips were dry, that she didn't drink anything, and that her mom carefully applied some lip balm. Amanda lay on her side, propped up on pillows, a nasal cannula delivering oxygen with a soft whir. Her parents lay in bed too — one on either side of her. Nobody spoke to me or looked at me, so I left the room.

If Amanda's life was a novel, I was a minor character — a character without lines. I sat at the nurse's station, wondering what I could do for her. My pager went off all night, calling me to other rooms and other patients, but I kept returning to the desk outside Amanda's room. "Do you think they need me?"

Amanda's nurse shook her head. "Best to leave them alone."

It was torture not to go in the room. Shouldn't I know the patient whose final event note I was to write? Shouldn't there be a moment of connection? Well, I had brought her a cup of water. Somehow that made me feel better.

I checked on Amanda twice more. The first time, she was cuddling with her mother. The second time, she appeared to be asleep. An hour or two later, her nurse called me. "I think she passed," she said. She was crying. Another nurse hugged her. I stood awkwardly, my hands in the pockets of my white coat. "Go on in," she said. "You have to pronounce her."

So that was my job — to listen to Amanda's quiet chest and confirm that she was gone. I put my stethoscope over her heart and listened for a long time. When I looked up, both parents were watching me. It was a strange moment, the three of us in the room with Amanda. I opened my mouth to speak, but they cut me off. They reached for each other. And that was the end of the story.

From Amanda, I learned Rule Number Three: *Family first*. I don't think her parents remember me. They probably remember Sam and their favorite nurse. I was just the one with the stethoscope, at the end — an extra in Amanda's story and the story of her family.

But in my own story, Amanda is a prominent figure. Because of her, I learned Rule Number Four: *12 hours is just the beginning*. Because I still think about Amanda Lopez, and it's five years later.

DON'T GIVE UP. The last rule, Rule Number Five. It's weeks later, and I am back in the ER with another medical student, telling him what I like about my job. The level of acuity, the interesting cases, the varied age groups. The many dramas, big and small, that come through my door each day. The medical student plans to go into general pediatrics because, he says, he likes the continuity of care. He wants to get to know his patients.

I defend my specialty. Children with respiratory illness often come back for a "resp check"—a second visit—and babies with fevers commonly are brought back to the ER for a follow-up visit as well. If we put in stitches, we usually take them out. I enjoy these reunions, the familiar faces, the "How are you doing?"

And even though there are many patients we never see again, I tell the student, *don't give up.* After all, a lot can be accomplished in just a few hours. Parties start and end. Entire weather systems change. Shakespeare's plays are just hours long, and think of all that happens there—people fall in love, wage war, return from exile. Kingdoms fall.

And, can you believe it? That same day, I bump into the grandmother at the end of my shift. We are both in the lobby, trying to exit the hospital through the revolving door. There are several people ahead of us, and we wait awkwardly together.

Finally, she nods at me.

"The kids?" I ask, looking around. She tells me she is here alone, visiting a sick relative.

"How are they?"

"*Malcriados.*" Poorly behaved.

"I'm sorry…" I begin.

She enters the revolving door, waving away my apology. "The woman came from ACS, she checked the house, she talked to us—and she left. She saw we were good people."

"I try to treat every family the same," I say, defending myself as I stumble through the door behind her.

She stands and faces me in the bright sunlight. Then, she surprises me. "You did the right thing," she says. "If somebody had done that for my brother and me when we were young, it might have saved his life." And just like that, she strides off in her thick heels. The whole conversation is two minutes from start to finish — about as long as it takes to adjust to the winter light, shake my head, and watch her disappear down the broad avenue.

Shifting Sands

Perri Klass, MD

For drama's sake, this story should start, "It was the coldest night of the year in Boston." Poetic license aside, it was a frigid January night, and I decided to splurge on the overpriced parking right near Symphony Hall. Now, I am not usually the symphony goer in my family; I am the parent who stays home with the kids so their father can enjoy his single Boston Symphony Orchestra subscription. This was a special treat: we had a babysitter, and Larry and I were meeting at Symphony Hall.

But my mind was not on music. I was in the middle of what we used to call a "social service code." Two evenings earlier, I had seen one of my regular patients, a three-month-old boy, for a checkup. I had treated his rather severe diaper rash, weighed and measured him — and worried. Because his mother seemed kind of stressed, kind of marginal, kind of over the edge. I knew some of her story: housing problems and homeless shelters, money problems, and legal problems. I had already invoked domestic violence services, family support services, patient advocate services, and the emergency clothing pantry. And, of course, the Department of Social Services. There was an open DSS case on the baby, and I had spoken many times with the DSS worker.

At the end of that visit, I told the mother that I was worried. She had run out of money and supplies from the Women, Infants, and Children program and was feeding the baby out of a big can of powdered elemental formula — nothing that would harm him, but something that must have been prescribed for some other baby with a digestive problem and come her way through her mysterious network of shadowy friends. The baby, who was usually dressed immaculately in outfits with matching socks and coordinated caps, looked scruffy and bedraggled. And the mother seemed…off somehow, all over the place, overwhelmed and disoriented.

It's hard to put into words the feeling she gave me — that's why I reach for these vague expressions of dislocation and discomfort. Or I could express it in jargon — she seemed "inappropriate"; she was showing "poor judgment." Whatever was going on in this family's life, I knew it wasn't good. When I asked about it, she shook her head and hinted darkly at disasters and betrayals. "But I've been praying a lot," she said.

So I told her I would call DSS in the morning, and she flinched. She felt judged and found guilty and perhaps betrayed yet again. "So they can help you," I said. "So they can make sure you have food for yourself and the baby and help straighten out your housing."

She and the baby went home (in a taxi, with a voucher from the health center), and in the morning I called her DSS worker and, as we say, expressed my concerns. "I feel strongly that this family needs more services," I said and listed some: parenting classes, medical and mental health evaluations for the mother, maybe an emergency stabilization team.

The next afternoon, before the concert, I was paged by DSS. Apparently, after the taxi took them home from the clinic, the mother had called a friend to come stay with the baby and had gone off — no one knew where — in search of food and money. And after some changes in baby-sitter, there had been some kind of crisis — someone who didn't want to stay or didn't know when the mother was coming back called the DSS hotline. DSS decided to take the baby into emergency custody and told the babysitter to wait there for the workers, but the babysitter panicked.

Or maybe the mother got home and panicked — nobody knew exactly. But when DSS got to the apartment, there was no one there. No babysitter, no mother, no three-month-old. Just an unlocked door, an empty apartment, and signs of a hasty departure.

I left word at the health center that if the mother called, DSS was to be informed at once. I called the apartment a couple of times, but no one answered.

And then it was time for the concert. As I parked my car, paid my $20, and walked out into the painfully cold air, I was thinking, melodramatically, *the coldest night of the year and that baby is out there someplace.* I thought about the gap between my own life and my patients' lives — if I had just handed the mother the $20 I was blowing on parking, she could have bought formula and food and not gone chasing off on some complicated avenue of her precarious life.

Then, the concert. As the non-symphony goer, I had very little idea what to expect; Berlioz, a bicentennial celebration of his birth, *L'Enfance du Christ*, a 19th-century oratorio, Larry said. Famous for its tenderness as the story of Christ's birth, for its chorus of shepherds saying goodbye as the Holy Family sets off on the flight into Egypt. We took our seats in Symphony Hall — which was warm, bright, beautiful, and extraordinarily civilized after our short dashes through the freezing evening — and watched the orchestra tune up, watched the chorus file onto the stage, applauded the conductor. I was obsessively rerunning in my mind the scenario of what I should have done two nights earlier, how I could have avoided this whole mess.

They kept the house lights on so we could follow along in the libretto.

L'Enfance du Christ starts with Herod's dream, an aria

in which the king is tortured by thoughts that a baby will undo him: *Oh the wretchedness of kings! To rule yet not to live, to mete out laws to all, yet to long to follow the goatherd into the heart of the woods!* And he orders the slaughter of all the newborn children.

I could pay attention. But the combination of the music and the words, the sitting still and listening, brought up with sudden and harsh force all the worst, most melodramatic tabloid images of where that baby might be. A three-month-old out there on the cold streets, his mother ducking into doorways when the wind blasted, dragging him around corners if a siren sounded. Would she have dressed him warmly enough? Would she understand how quickly a baby could freeze? Was she unhinged by the thought of people coming to take away her child or by this last set of betrayals — me calling to complain about her, the babysitter calling to report her? In my music-enhanced imagination, I saw her moving toward some decision point — toward a bridge, perhaps, the baby in her arms. I saw old-movie black-and-white shadows, gloomy Victorian paintings of disgraced or despondent women. I saw death and disaster and destruction.

And, of course, I saw myself as responsible. Interestingly, I was managing to blame myself along two completely different tracks, in both cases putting myself at the center of the story. In one version, I was wrong to have called DSS at all: Why hadn't I dealt with the problems of the moment, handed the woman $20 for formula, given her a pep talk about how hard she was trying, promised more help in the morning, and sent her home feeling supported? I had undermined her and invoked the powers of the state when all she needed was some cash and a sense that there was someone on her side. But I didn't really believe this, though the idea of handing her $20 had taken on a certain irresistible appeal ever since I'd parked my car.

Mostly, I blamed myself in the other direction, holding this doublethink quite comfortably in my mind: Why on earth had I let her take that little baby home two nights ago? Wasn't there enough evidence that things were falling apart, that the child was at risk? I flip-flopped from the image of handing her the $20 and patting her shoulder to a different, fiercer scenario: call the security guard, station him outside the exam room, call the DSS emergency hotline…

Where was the mother? Where was the baby? I had left my beeper in the car and turned off my cell phone. I could picture the beeper chirping away in the ice-cold car. Why had I ever invoked DSS; why hadn't I just sent her home encouraged? How could I have let her take that baby home; why hadn't I called the hotline there and then?

And it was so cold out. The chorus of shepherds sang their farewell, and Jesus, Mary, and Joseph were journeying through the desert: *For three days, despite the hot winds, they journeyed through the shifting sands.* And the city outside seemed to me right then like a frozen desert, barren and hostile to life. And yet there I was, sitting in a glorious building, rich with light and music, voices and instruments. A building and a moment, testament, if anything could be, to the glory of cities and of group human enterprise.

In the oratorio, the weary family comes to a city. Mary sings, *In this immense town the roar and bustle of the hurrying crowds! Joseph, I'm frightened…I can't go on…* Joseph knocks first on one door and then on another, begging for shelter, rest, and food, only to be reviled by the chorus: "Get away, vile Hebrews! Egyptian people have nothing to do with tramps and lepers!"

Had I somehow helped to turn this little family away, to launch it into a world of closed doors, hostile winds, and, at least figuratively, shifting sands? When I closed my eyes, the images I saw were appropriately biblical and desert-themed, but they flickered every so often into a more modern, cold-climate picture: a woman, not warmly enough dressed, hurrying down a dark Boston street, clutching an infant car seat by its handle, hiding from everyone who might try to take her baby away. She tried so hard to be a conscientious mother; she had a car seat, I knew, although she had no car.

I didn't actually start crying until the last scene, when Joseph knocked on the Ishmaelite's door and the family was welcomed in and comforted. I'm not sure exactly why I was crying. Maybe it was at the possibility of help and kindness coming out of bleakness and despair for an individual baby, an individual family, a door opening just when the whole town seemed closed. Or maybe it was at some confused, sentimental geopolitical thought: as the householder sang, *Don't be afraid; the children of Ishmael are brothers of the children of Israel,* it occurred to me that in this musical fantasy, one charitable home enclosed Jews, the child Jesus, and those who would later be Muslims — a 19th-century French version of a human peaceable kingdom. I was, I suppose, a little overwrought.

Whomever I was crying for — myself, my patient, or the world — the music ended, and I wiped my eyes, made the cold dash back to my car, and went home and worried.

In the morning, of course, it all turned out all right. There had been misunderstandings and miscommunications — mother and baby had been safe and warm inside all night, the mother having conscientiously left messages on various official answering machines. If it hadn't all been a triumph of good maternal judgment, neither had it been egregious neglect or avoidance of the authorities.

There were still, as we say, multiple issues. The family was still, as we say, of great concern. But both mother and baby were okay. I probably wouldn't be telling this story if they hadn't been.

But, of course, their story doesn't end there. It goes on, in this real city in which they live, which is not the same city I know, with complications and arrangements and contingencies that I can't even guess, with catastrophes and threats and just getting by. I see little bits, try to help patch services together, and worry that it will again fall to me to sit in judgment. They manage, but only just. There are moments of grace and moments of safety, moments of shelter and moments of comfort, and all of that is real. But for this mother and baby, I fear, the wilderness is also real, and the wilderness is infinite.

THE MISSING PIECE

Huy Quang Nguyen, MD

"**D**R. HUY, WE'VE TRIED everything. What should we do?" Thuy's mother pleaded with me.

At that moment, as if directed in concert, the chorus of crying children in other exam rooms quieted. The clack-clack tapping of Thuy's plastic bottle on my desk stopped. Even the purring of the desktop computer fan switched off. The universe paused and waited for me to expound.

I pulled at my collar. I frowned and noted the sweat condensing in my armpits. Then I did what any experienced physician would do when he does not have the faintest clue.

I stalled.

Perhaps if given sufficient space and time, I thought, the answer might rise up out of the humid air. I woke up the computer and began pulling up Thuy's growth charts. I adjusted my seat. I reviewed the details again in my mind.

Thuy was an 18-month-old girl who was born healthy and full-term at a local Boston hospital. She was the first child to her 20-something-year-old parents, who had immigrated to the United States from Vietnam six years ago.

For the first six months of life, she had fattened through a regimen of nursing and liberal formula supplementation. Her weight growth curve described a steep mountain, peaking at the 95th percentile at seven months of age. And then, while all of the normative percentile curves continued in a smooth upward arc, Thuy's weight growth curve plateaued. Even as her length and head circumference growth curves rose normally, her weight growth curve stubbornly stayed flat. Over time, it gradually crossed the 50th, and then the 25th, and finally, the 10th percentile. Thuy was getting taller, but she was not gaining any weight.

At 18 months old, she weighed only 21 pounds, the average weight of a 12-month-old child. She had a wizened appearance, with thin arms and legs, a bony chest, a gaunt mouselike face, and thin, sparse hair. In spite of her lack of bulk, Thuy's motor and language development were roughly age-appropriate. Earlier during the visit, when I approached to examine her, she screeched, gripped her mother tightly, and deftly avoided the touch of my stethoscope, just as any of my hardier toddler patients would.

In our office library, all of the pediatric textbooks dedicated a chapter to Thuy's condition, aptly called "failure to thrive." Symmetric failure to thrive, characterized by a flattening of the weight, length, and head circumference growth curves, has a dizzyingly long list of potential causes, from inborn genetic mutations to acquired hormonal imbalances. Failure to thrive primarily affecting weight, however, such as in Thuy's case, almost always has a psychosocial problem at its root. These problems include parental neglect, emotional deprivation, poverty, and malnutrition.

It did not make any sense.

Thuy's parents both had steady jobs. Her father owned a small hardwood floor refinishing company. Her mother, Ha, worked as a manicurist in one of the many neighborhood nail salons. Thuy's parents had even managed to save enough money to buy a modest house. They had many family supports in place. Thuy's maternal grandparents often cared for her during the day. The entire extended family visibly doted on the little girl and described spending hours feeding her meticulously prepared Vietnamese dishes traditionally offered to toddlers.

I looked up from the computer at Ha. She was staring at me, waiting for my response, eyes full of desperation. The room was still quiet, but now the silence seemed compressed into the instant before a revelatory big bang. By now, the sweat was dripping down my flanks.

I opened my mouth to speak, but nothing happened.

I still did not have the answer.

Instead, I ordered laboratory tests to exclude the most common disease-related causes for failure to thrive. Then I arranged for Thuy and her mother to follow up with me in one month.

Much later that day, I found myself lying in bed, thinking about my predicament. Five years ago, when I returned to Boston after finishing my pediatric residency training in Seattle, I knew that I would be serving an inner-city community. What I did not foresee, however, was that my patient panel would be largely comprised of newly immigrated Vietnamese families.

These Vietnamese parents brought their children to me to be treated, hoping and expecting to find a pediatrician with a familiar Vietnamese name and a common Vietnamese experience. They were in for a surprise. Unlike many of the other, older Vietnamese physicians in the area, who had been educated and trained in Vietnam, I was a relatively young physician, not quite fluent in Vietnamese, who had lived nearly all of his 35 years in the United States.

My family arrived in the United States in 1975 as refugees from the Vietnam War. My parents were eager for their children to learn English first and foremost. They believed that early acculturation was the price of access to America's opportunity. Growing up with very few Vietnamese families living nearby, eager to succeed in the classroom and in the playground, I became fluent not just in English but also in the customs and mores of American society. While I share a common heritage with my Vietnamese patients, whenever I struggle to communicate with them, I often feel our kinship ends there, on the shores of a country half a world away.

Unable to sleep, I was nagged by the feeling that Thuy's case was one of those situations. As strange as it seemed, her story was not unique. In fact, the thin 18-month-old seemed nearly identical to many other Vietnamese toddlers I treated. All were lovingly cared for by appropriately anxious parents, yet all began to fail to thrive in their sixth to ninth month of life. The more I tried to fit the details of these cases into those "classic" psychosocial failure to thrive cases I read about in textbooks, however, the more obscure the answer seemed. The clues were all there in front of me, but the pieces did not fit together. What was I missing? If the solution were embedded in the Vietnamese identity of these families, did I, with my altogether different immigrant experience, have any chance of finding it?

It was then, in the depths of my self-doubt, that I experienced the beginnings of hope. I remembered seeing a small, black-and-white picture of a gaunt, wispy-haired 15-month-old boy holding a cardboard placard with white chalk numbers on it. Not more than a mug shot, this refugee identification picture is the earliest picture of me that survived my family's flight from Vietnam. In the image of this undernourished Vietnamese child, I saw the face of my failure-to-thrive patient, Thuy. If the boy in that picture was in fact me, then I shared much more with my Vietnamese patients than I thought. Maybe it was not the body of medical knowledge I had mastered but, instead, the life I had lived that would lift me out of my predicament.

Thuy returned a month later with her mother, Ha. I reviewed all of the normal blood test results, which ruled out so-called organic causes of failure to thrive. As I searched for the missing puzzle piece, I asked Ha to describe what it was like to feed Thuy.

"Thuy doesn't want to eat," replied Ha, sighing. "I offer her three meals a day, but it's so hard to feed her. We give her rice soup because we are afraid she'll choke on foods that she has to chew. I spend a lot of time making the rice soup with broth steeped from boiled pork bones. I skim off all of the fat that rises to the surface of the broth, because the fat is too 'hot' and difficult to digest for Thuy's immature stomach. Thuy will eat the first few bites readily, but then refuses to open her mouth to take the spoon I offer her."

Ha wrung her hands in frustration.

"Because of this struggle to feed her, meals often take an hour long," she continued. "And she won't even take her bottle of whole milk as much as she used to. Sometimes we even have to use a syringe to squirt the rice soup or milk into her mouth."

"But Thuy is 18 months old already," I pointed out. "Do you ever let her feed herself?"

"No. She would make too much of a mess," Ha

replied. "Besides, if we don't feed her ourselves, we feel guilty that we're not doing enough to help her to gain weight and grow. After all, she's just a baby."

With this emotional response, Thuy's mother revealed to me the solution. When Ha and I looked at Thuy, in effect we saw two different children. Through the eyes of my pediatric training based on Western models of child development, up until this point, I had been seeing an 18-month-old toddler who had graduated from infancy. I had envisioned Thuy embarking on a new independence. I had expected her behavior to be driven by a desire for self-mastery of new skills such as running, climbing, talking, self-feeding, self-dressing, and, soon, toileting. Thuy's mother, however, was informed by a different paradigm of child development based on Vietnamese cultural tradition. In Vietnam, infancy is traditionally thought to extend until two years old. According to common Vietnamese customs, Thuy, at 18 months old, was still too young to tolerate foods commonly eaten by adults. For this reason, as her staple diet, Thuy's parents continued to feed her a watery rice soup that was very low in caloric density.

Because they still considered her to be an infant, Thuy's family continued to spoon-feed her and did not allow her to feed herself. This traditional parent-centered model led them to disregard Thuy's satiety cues. When Thuy turned her face away or refused to open her mouth to take the spoon, they redoubled their efforts to persuade her to open up. Sometimes they resorted to using a syringe to squirt rice soup or milk in through the little girl's pursed lips.

Thuy's family's overwhelming anxiety about her weight stemmed from their own experience in Vietnam. Of the 20 countries that account for the majority of the world's undernourished children, Vietnam ranks among the most affected. Young children who do not gain weight eventually develop stunting, a reduction in height due to undernutrition. In Vietnam, the prevalence of stunting exceeds 40 percent. Thuy's family's fears, however, resulted in overly aggressive feeding practices. For Thuy, eating had become an unpleasant activity during which she felt pressured and besieged. She was beginning to develop an aversion to eating.

As the pieces of the puzzle fell in place, I realized that successfully treating Thuy's failure to thrive and the similar problem experienced by many of my other young Vietnamese patients could not be solved with a prescription. Perhaps, too, attempting to alter how Thuy's parents fundamentally perceived their 18-month-old daughter was an impossible cultural minefield. As I noted Ha's exasperated expression and her exhausted posture, however, there was one thing of which I was certain. Ha's battles with her daughter around the dinner table were not only ineffective, they were also unsustainable. And even if I did not have the complete answer, the image of that little refugee boy reassured me. At least now I knew how to begin the conversation.

Once she finished with her story, Thuy's mother again implored me.

"Dr. Huy, we've tried everything. What should we do?"

This time, within that quiet space between her question and my answer, a Vietnamese proverb I had heard many times came into my mind:

"To appreciate me, you must appreciate the journey I have taken to come here."

That was what I needed to do. When faced with a confusing clinical puzzle, consider the patient's cultural identity, literally shaped by the journey of a lifetime. In this case, I found the missing piece in the most unexpected of places, along the path of my own journey.

Of course, I thought. How could I forget? Smiling, I shut off the computer. Turning to look at the little girl and her mother, I began.

"I think I can help."

Double-Talk

Eileen Costello, MD

THERE ARE PLENTY of secrets in primary care. With each passing year, I am aware of more of them. The children who don't know that their dad isn't really their dad; the mom whose husband doesn't know she was married before; the histories of abuse that people keep to themselves out of a sense of shame and a perceived need to protect their families. Sometimes the secrets are brought to light by some unexpected stress in the family. Then, the fact that I was already in on them puts me in a terrible position with regard to maintaining the trust of the various members of the family. I then repeat the mantra: *the child is my patient, the child is my patient, the child is my patient.*

The secrets are one of the many aspects of practicing pediatrics for which medical school and residency training didn't prepare me. I wasn't prepared for some of the obvious things that we all complain about, such as the finances, the hiring of staff, keeping the place running smoothly, and being accessible to our patients and their families. But the not-so-obvious things are what make it interesting. I am frequently perplexed in the exam room, trying to figure out who knows what in the patient's family, trying to respect the privacy of the patients to the extent that is reasonable, while doing my job of providing care. The practice I work in is an urban (some might say "inner-city") health center with a remarkably diverse patient population. My colleagues and I spend a fair amount of time thinking about the different expectations that our patients' families have for their encounters with us.

I recently saw a 12-year-old patient who came in with her mom. On the encounter form outside the exam room, the reason for the visit was given as "sore throat." Excellent, I thought, a quick visit; this would help me catch up with the folks in the waiting room, some of whom were giving me the evil eye when they could catch my glance. As I entered the room, the mom asked if she could speak to me privately. Okay, not a sore throat, I figured, wondering what would come next. I did not know this mom; her daughter was usually seen by one of my colleagues. She told me her daughter had developed a new behavior over the last few months. She was making sounds with her throat and twitching her face and did not seem to be aware of it. She had a brother close to her age who was embarrassed by this, and he made fun of her the way only a close sibling can. The mom was worried that the girl's behavior represented some kind of possession by an evil force. The stunning thing, however, was that she wanted me to talk to her daughter as if this was something *I* was noticing coincidentally and to try and open a conversation about it. I was to go along with the charade that her mom was unaware of this behavior, that it was just this interesting thing I happened to notice, and what did she think it was all about? The mom wanted me to *make it go away*, but I was not to make any recommendations about medicines, because she was opposed to the use of medications in children. Pretty tall orders.

I could not even imagine what life was like for this poor 12-year-old girl who, judging by this history, had Tourette's syndrome. Kids are cruel, and children with Tourette's are frequently on the receiving end of brutal teasing and bullying. The so-called zero tolerance for bullying provides them little protection, as the bullying is often so subtle that the adults miss it completely. So her brother was teasing her, and the adults in her family couldn't even talk about the issue.

When I walked into the room, the daughter told me she didn't know why she was there, that her mom had made this appointment and brought her in. This is definitely not the first time I've had a parent make an appointment and tell the child it was for something other than the real reason the parent wanted the child to be seen.

Sometimes we are asked to get a urine specimen, looking for drugs of abuse in the urine, without letting the teenager know that's what we are doing. That is so egregious that most of us just won't do it without engaging the patient in a conversation about the parent's concerns. Or sometimes the patient makes the appointment but doesn't give the real reason: a teenage girl will make an appointment for something like a "sore toe," when in fact she hasn't had a period for three months. It happens all the time. The problem is, how do you know how much time to allot to the visit, and how do you explain to the parents and their kids in the waiting room, who dutifully made their appointments months ago and showed up on time, why you are running overtime yet again?

In this case, the girl's symptoms were so profound that it was breathtaking that the family hadn't found a way to talk about them. While her symptoms were involuntary, she was certainly aware of them, and being in an office with a doctor heightened her anxiety and increased the twitching. She was relieved when I asked her about her symptoms, told her I had seen kids like her before, and said that we could probably help her. Her mom was also relieved that a conversation had been started. I wondered what would happen when they left. I made referrals for appointments with specialists. Would they keep them? Would they be able to talk about the problem? Would the girl ask her mom why she hadn't mentioned it, or would she believe that her mom really didn't notice? What about her brother?

Another teenager and her mom showed up a couple of weeks ago. This mom was worried that her daughter's periods had stopped. She wanted a medical evaluation. *I* knew the daughter was on her third round of Depo-Provera for contraception, which often halts periods altogether. I had started her on it myself, proud of her for taking control of her reproductive life. Sometimes I think providing contraception for sexually active teenagers is the single most important thing we as pediatricians do for our patients, next to immunizations. I was also aware, however, that her mom was not in the loop. The patient had told me her mother would be so angry and upset if she knew her daughter was having sex that she would throw her out of the house. We are legally obligated to provide confidential care to adolescents seeking contraception, and since she was 16, I had less of the am-I-doing-the-right-thing? anxiety I have with a 13- or 14-year-old.

I asked the mom to provide us with some privacy for a physical exam, but she refused. So I closed the curtain separating the exam table from the rest of the room and proceeded to examine my patient. She used sign language, her finger across her throat, to communicate to me that she would be dead meat if I let her mother in on the real reason she wasn't having periods anymore. I opened the curtain after the exam and sat down to explain to the mom that this happens sometimes in teenagers, which is true; that at this moment we could probably wait and watch and that I would see her again in another month. As they left, I found myself wondering whether the mom knew exactly what was going on but somehow needed her daughter to believe that she didn't. If she did know, then she knew that I knew but was not at liberty to tell her, and that her daughter obviously knew that I knew and that she didn't. On the other hand, if the mom really *didn't* know, then she was in the dark; the daughter and I knew something that the mom didn't. Yes, the teenager was my patient, not her mother, but as a mother of teenagers myself, I often find myself in that sticky place where I *want* the parents to know what is going on with their son or daughter. It's just kind of creepy, feeling that I am playing tricks on the parents who are paying the bills and bringing the kids to their doctor for some sound advice.

In another case, a five-year-old boy who had had a first-time seizure came in with his mom to review the events of his emergency room evaluation and talk about referral to a neurologist. I had known this little guy his entire life and felt quite connected to his mom, who had a couple of other kids. I had met their dad a few times, but it was almost always the mom who brought the kids in for their visits with me. As we talked, I asked the usual family history questions: Has anyone in the family ever had a seizure? Parents, siblings, cousins, grandparents? It's very striking how a family history of a medical condition can come to light when a child in the family has a new-onset medical problem. I am particularly interested in the genetic basis for the many things that ail children and probably ask about family history more than is typical. On many occasions, a parent has discovered that yes, there is relevant family medical history, but no one had ever thought it was relevant until now.

In the case of my little boy with a new-onset seizure, I was surprised to learn from the mom that the child's dad had been adopted — and the family history on his side was unknown. I looked into the record to discover a long list of medical complaints among the dad's siblings. When I asked the mom about this, she volunteered that her husband did not know that he was adopted — that his mother had told her, his wife, but that he himself didn't know and neither did their children. The family had decided that this was best for him, that he would be too upset if he knew. The idea of not telling relatives a vital piece of information under the guise of "protecting" them is familiar to me. I was raised with this idea, in my Irish-Catholic family, keeping a secret from the person who most needs the information, while everyone around that person is in the know.

My usual strategy is to do what I feel necessary to take care of my primary care patients and to let the family know, over time, that secrets are almost never a great idea. That's the best thing about the primary care relationship: it evolves over time. If the parents stick it out with me over their child's life, that can last for 20 years. That's a lot of time to try and make things right, to get everything clear, and to make referrals to people who might help a family figure these things out. In the meantime, we work together. I can only work with what I know, not with what I don't know.

Whenever possible, I let families know my own opinion about these types of secrets. With some, I can be pretty clear. I can say, "This is nuts! Have you really thought about this? This isn't healthy for your kids. Lots more damage will be done if this secret continues to be kept." Often I tell the teenagers that it's pretty unlikely their parents are as in the dark as they like to think. Parents were teenagers too, after all. Most primary care visits do not require a review of what's known and what isn't among various family members. But it comes up often enough, and raises all types of interesting questions. Do I note my new information in the medical record? Is it appropriate for me to make a notation about the adopted dad, if he himself doesn't know? Or do I try to file it somewhere or make a cryptic notation to myself that only I will understand? Sometimes I wonder how often I am the one who doesn't know something, how often some critical piece of history is not told to me, how often I am working in the dark.

Paula's Story

Mariana Glusman, MD

I STARTED SEEING PAULA almost ten years ago. She was one of my first patients as an attending (just so you don't think I'm that old). She was referred to me from the NICU, a six-month-old, former 24-week preemie who had had a remarkably uncomplicated course for her gestational age. Her main issue at that time was feeding and growing, and she had been discharged on nasogastric feeds, formula pumped down into her stomach through a thin tube that passed through her nostril and then down her esophagus. She was tiny, and so was her mom, a four-foot-nine Mexican woman who was probably in her late 30s but looked much older than that.

I started with the history. I am bilingual and bicultural, so language was not an issue for me. The mom was relieved to have a Spanish-speaking doctor. But I did not have a discharge summary from the hospital, and she was only able to tell me that Paula was born four months early, that she had a tube in her throat for a long time, that she had been given lots of medicines and had lots of studies done, that the baby had been discharged the week before, and that at night and during the day she hooked the baby up to the machine to feed her. She did bring a list of her medicines and follow-up appointments, and she said that things were fine since they had been home.

Just sorting this out took more time than I had, so I went on to the physical exam. I picked Paula up from her mother's lap to help the mom place her on the exam table, and the first thing that the mother said to me was, "Do you know how to hold a baby?" Well, I felt very insulted. Of course I know how to hold a baby! I had two kids of my own, and I had just finished three years of pediatric residency. I examined the baby, reinforced the plan of care as best I could, and had them return in one week for a weight check. In the meantime, I could get the records from the NICU.

In her first two years I saw Paula all the time — for weight gain issues, for multiple viral infections, for chronic lung disease, developmental delays — the usual preemie stuff. And she quickly became one of my least favorite patients. Despite the fact that there was no language barrier (if I had had to see her mom with a translator, I might have shot myself), each visit took forever. I was very frustrated with the mom's noncompliance. It seemed that I went over the same issues every time. I can't tell you how many times I wrote in her chart, "discussed AGAIN [underlined three times in frustration] the importance of taking Flovent EVERY DAY!" Each time, the mom would nod and act as if it was the first time I'd ever said it. She would also fail to keep her appointments with the specialists. But she did keep coming to see me. Once, she said that she didn't want to give Paula medicine every day because she did not want her to get hooked on it. On occasion, I know that she took her to a *curandero* (folk healer).

As time went by, I got to know Paula's mom better. She grew up in a village in Mexico. She attended first grade only, because a girl at the school was raped and her dad did not allow her to go to school anymore. She had two grown children in Mexico. She had been in the United States for only a couple of years. She was now married to a younger man (Paula's father), and they had a cart and sold corn in the streets in their Mexican neighborhood. They earned very little but sent money every month to her husband's mother in Mexico. I also learned that Paula's dad was an alcoholic, and I have a feeling there was some domestic violence at the time (though I have to admit that I never directly asked). Paula's mom would take the corn cart in her van and drive to where she was going to sell the corn. She would park the car within view, and Paula would stay in the car while her mom worked. They lived and worked in a high-crime neighborhood. She told me that sometimes she was afraid and that she had been in the middle of gang shootings.

A couple of years ago, Paula's mom told me she had gone to visit her family in Mexico. I asked her how she did it, since I knew that she was in the country illegally. She had told me that it costs about $2,000 to get into the United States (imagine how much corn that is!). The first time she tried, she had to crawl on her hands and knees through a pipe to cross the border. Unfortunately, she was caught and sent back. Then she paid some more to get false papers. She memorized everything about her new identity, and this time she passed all the questioning by immigration and was allowed back in. "After the officer finished his questions, I got up and left. I was so nervous. I never looked back." Knowing that she had only finished first grade, I asked her how she had been able to keep all the documents straight. She told me that she had taught herself how to read. "Do you want me to show you?" she asked. I told her no, that I believed her, but she pulled out a little book from her bag that looked like a Bible. She had gotten this book from Al-Anon and carried it with her always. She started to read aloud in a monotone, and then she paused, smiling. "See these little dots on the page?" she asked. "They tell you when one sentence ends and the next one begins."

Paula is one of my favorite patients now, and I have the utmost respect for her mom. What incredible strength and courage! As I think back on how frustrated I felt with her, I realize that, fresh out of residency, I had no idea about how difficult it really was, in the context of her life, for her to follow the advice I gave her. I had blamed her for being "noncompliant" and for "failing" her follow-up appointments. I see now that the instructions that I thought were perfectly clear were not (for example, "take two puffs twice a day") and that going to follow-up specialty visits requires many steps, from making the appointment, to finding the clinic, to filling out forms, to understanding what the doctors are saying, to trusting their recommendations.

I am now much more patient with families. I think of "adherence" rather than "compliance." I have become more knowledgeable about health literacy and health disparities and the barriers that families face, and I have changed my practice to use plain language and elicit patient understanding. Paula is doing remarkably well for being a former 24-week preemie, and ten years later, I am a better doctor because of her — and her mom.

There's a
Bug in Your Head

Patrick McDonald, MD, MHSC, FRCSC

BECAUSE I WAS BORN, raised, and educated in Toronto, my exposure to First Nations people and cultures was limited to what little attention was paid them by the mainstream media and the educational system. When I became an intern and resident in a downtown hospital, the familiar stereotypes were reinforced by encounters with homeless adult Natives, many with substance abuse problems. I confess to not giving aboriginal issues in medicine and in Canada much thought.

All that changed when I moved to Winnipeg to practice as a pediatric neurosurgeon at Winnipeg Children's

Hospital. Winnipeg has a larger aboriginal population than any other major city in Canada, and First Nations people make a significant contribution to its cultural and artistic vibrancy. For the first time in my career, I encountered First Nations children on a daily basis.

One of my new patients was a seven-year-old boy named Timmy. He lived on a remote reserve several hours from Winnipeg, accessible only by air. Timmy had suffered headaches for a few weeks and was starting to develop weakness in his left arm and leg. CT and MRI scans revealed a large cystic tumor in his upper brainstem extending into his right thalamus. Despite his headaches, Timmy was a happy, active child. He spoke Oji-Cree and very little English, and he seemed to want nothing to do with me until I showed him I could wiggle my nose just like he could.

I met with Timmy's mother to explain the nature of Timmy's brain tumor, propose surgery, and discuss the potential risks and expected recovery time. Parents usually react to a talk like this with a mixture of fear, anger, and grief. They often question why this happened to their child. But for the most part, Timmy's mom seemed unconcerned with these issues. Her questions threw me off guard. They didn't have hot water in their small house on the reserve — could I help them get it? What about an indoor toilet? As a matter of fact, maybe I could write to the authorities and stress that they needed a new house altogether.

My first reaction was disbelief — this woman seemed

more concerned about material things than the health of her son. But over the next days and weeks, I began to understand that these were legitimate questions from a woman anxious not just about the welfare of her sick child (though she clearly was deeply worried about this) but also about the welfare of her entire family. Her questions implied a fear of being unable to care adequately for a child who could be quite sick for a long time in conditions where it was hard enough to raise healthy children.

When it came time to officially get consent for the proposed surgery, a meeting with the family was arranged. I like to meet with parents and one or two other close relatives or friends (and the child, if he or she is old enough). I typically refuse requests to meet with large groups of people — I find that too many different people asking questions tends to confuse things. In this case, though, I quickly realized that the process of obtaining consent would not be typical.

When I entered, aunts, uncles, brothers, sisters, and parents crowded the room. An older woman sat in the far corner, saying nothing but listening intently throughout the encounter. Introductions were made, and I began with my usual description of the clinical picture, proposed intervention, alternatives, risks, and probable outcomes. I was then peppered with questions: Would Timmy be okay? Would he be able to go back to school? Play outside? Fish? Had I ever done this type of surgery before?

I answered as best I could, and then something remarkable happened. Timmy's aunts, uncles, and mother all turned to the older woman in the corner of the room — Timmy's grandmother, who had not yet spoken — and asked, "What should we do?" She paused, then said: "We should go ahead with the surgery." That was it. No more questions — the decision had been made.

Later that day, I told his mother that Timmy should know what was going to happen. In a matter-of-fact way, she informed me they had already told him, "You have a bug in your head" — pronounced "munjuice" in Oji-Cree — "and the doctor is going to take it out." When I saw Timmy, he quickly pointed to his head, saying "munjuice" and smiled while wiggling his nose.

I've been in Winnipeg four years now, and the consent process I experienced with Timmy and his family has been repeated countless times with other First Nations families. It always includes extended family supporting the child and parents, with the wisdom of older members actively sought and respected. I am struck by the strength of the family unit — something not often mentioned in the mainstream media.

Timmy's tumor came out uneventfully. Fortunately, it was a benign brain tumor of childhood. The day after his surgery, Timmy pointed to his head and asked, "Munjuice?" He smiled when his mother looked at me and said, "No more munjuice."

THE GIFT OF SIGHT

Diego Chaves-Gnecco, MD, MPH

As on most Sunday mornings, my wife and I were attending our weekly Mass in Spanish. It was a beautiful day, and even inside the church we were able to see the light of the sun streaming through the stained-glass windows. Sitting in front of us was a family of three: a mother and two beautiful preschool-aged girls. I didn't remember seeing them before at the church or in the community. I was pretty sure about this, as I would have remembered what started to concern me then. One of the girls had severe esotropia (crossed eyes), and I wondered about the quality of her vision. She was not wearing glasses, and she came very close to her sister when interacting with her, as if she had trouble seeing.

Throughout the Mass, I struggled with what was appropriate for me to do in this situation. In my home country of Colombia, the Latino culture allows for our personal boundaries to be closer; our Latino culture is all about community. Here in my new home, the American culture is all about privacy and independence. Despite these differences in culture, I wondered how unusual it might be for someone to approach you to discuss your daughter's vision in church. Perhaps it would have been less awkward back at home in Colombia. Was it appropriate for me to talk to this lady about my concerns related to her daughter's vision, given that I was a stranger in an unusual environment?

I asked my wife for her opinion. I thought she would provide me with a reality check. But she said, "If you are concerned about this little girl's vision, talk to her mother; she will understand."

Still a bit uneasy due to the unusual circumstances, I approached the mother. I introduced myself and told her about the concerns that I had for her daughter. I told her that I was a resident at Children's Hospital of Pittsburgh of UPMC and that two years ago I had created the first bilingual/bicultural clinic in southwestern Pennsylvania: Salud Para Niños (Health for Children). I offered her my help to address my concerns about her daughter's vision. Mrs. García very politely declined my offer. She told me she already had seen her pediatrician and they had a referral for an eye doctor. I thanked her for her time and for sharing this with me, and left Mass feeling relieved. But

I could tell Mrs. García had not completely trusted me, and I was still uncertain whether her daughter's vision problems would be addressed.

Two weeks went by, and this time I was in the hospital in the middle of one of my ward rotations. I received a page from one of my colleagues asking me for help. They had a patient in the outpatient clinic with a skin injury, and they wanted to ensure that the discharge instructions in Spanish were given in a clear manner to the family. I came down to the Primary Care Center (our outpatient clinic) and was surprised to discover that the family that they were seeing was Mrs. García and her daughter, April. Mrs. García clearly remembered me from the church. I said hello to them and made a comment to the effect of, "After all, we are your pediatricians," to which she smiled and nodded her head. I took some time to make sure that they understood that April had to take an antibiotic four times a day for ten days, even if she was doing okay, and that if she had any fevers, pain, swelling, or purulent discharge, they had to let us know or come to our emergency room.

Once I was sure that they understood these instructions and had them repeat them back to me, I asked her if it was okay to talk to her about her daughter's vision. Mrs. García agreed. I told her that I was concerned about April's skin injury but that I was even more concerned about her vision. I told her that I understood that the visit was for a different concern, but I wanted to make sure that we addressed both, and that perhaps April's vision was even more important. She nodded again. After a pause, I asked her, "Did you make the appointment for the eye doctor?" Mrs. García blushed and proceeded in an earnest but calm manner to explain her problems. April had been seen by one of our residents several months earlier during a well child checkup. She was then referred to an ophthalmologist, but Mrs. García was not able to follow this recommendation because she didn't speak English and didn't know how or where she could make this appointment. She didn't know what to do about it. At this point, I realized that Mrs. García finally trusted me.

When I proposed the creation of our program, Salud Para Niños, I envisioned it as a "medical home" for our Hispanic/Latino community. One of the roles of medical homes is to help with referrals and assist with scheduling appointments. I told Mrs. García that I was going to help her with this appointment. A few days later, while completing a rotation at the pediatric intensive care unit, I read the ophthalmologist's note in our electronic medical records. He had seen April García in his clinic, and he was extremely concerned about April's presentation. She had a severe and unusual case of bilateral amblyopia (lazy eye, in both eyes). He had recommended that April use an eye patch (by patching one eye, the other eye is forced to develop and improve its vision), and he had also recommended a genetics consult, as April's unusual presentation had made him wonder about a genetic syndrome that might explain her symptoms. He had prescribed eyeglasses as well.

Almost immediately, I called Mrs. García. She told me that they had seen the ophthalmologist. I told her that I had read his note. I went on to ask her how she was doing with his recommendations for April. She told me that she understood how to do the eye patching, the reason for this, and the urgency of it. She had some questions about the genetics appointment, but the real roadblock this time was learning how to fill the prescription for April's eyeglasses, since she didn't speak English. I told her that I would help her with this. I called April's health insurance company and found an optician near her home. I also called the optician and explained the situation to him. I told him that Mrs. García was going to come with her prescription, that she didn't speak English, and that she desperately needed these glasses for her daughter. I also asked him to make sure that nothing but her insurance coverage was used, as we wanted to make sure they didn't end up with extra expenses or other complications. Somehow, the two managed to communicate with no words at all: the optician didn't speak Spanish, and Mrs. García didn't speak English. But Mrs. García filled the prescription, and April started wearing her glasses immediately.

I remember the first day I saw her in church with her new glasses. This time, she could probably see the beautiful sunlight streaming through the church's stained-glass windows. That day, I remembered why I had chosen to be a pediatrician—I knew I was able to make a difference in this family's life. April had received the gift of sight from her glasses—and also the gift of having had her needs met.

I felt that I, too, had received a gift of sight from April and her family. I could see, once again, my role as a pediatrician in our community: the Latino pediatrician who is part of the community he serves, who goes to church with his patients. My role in my adopted home.

It has been four years since then. April is still wearing her glasses all the time, though she needs some accommodations at school due to her vision problems. I am now the regular pediatrician for April, her sister, and her almost two-year-old brother. Mr. and Mrs. García recently asked me if I would like to be the girls' godfather for their baptism. I humbly accepted this great honor. I can say that I am the pediatrician of the Salud Para Niños community, which is also my community now too—something that makes me feel very proud.

In a recent meeting with the Allegheny County Department of Human Services, we were discussing starting a family support center for our community. The García family was there among other families with their children. We went around the table introducing ourselves. Because the idea of the project is mainly focused on families with children, the moderator asked us to say whether any of us had children ourselves. When it was my turn toward the end, I said, "My name is Diego Chaves-Gnecco, and I am a pediatrician in this community. And I don't have children yet, as my wife and I were recently married." Almost all of the families in the room interrupted to correct me: "Dr. Diego has six hundred children. Our children are his children."

Why?

Joy Marasco Neyhart, DO, FAAP

As a pediatrician in a remote part of Alaska, the riskiest part of my job by far is the care of a sick newborn. Although my pediatric residency included more neonatology than many other programs, I am not a neonatologist. There are times, however, when my training and skills are invaluable. There are also times, thankfully rare, when my training and skills still cannot save the life of a newborn. This is Rachel's story. It is no less painful for me now, over a year after her birth and — three short hours later — her death.

Rachel's mother had by all accounts a normal pregnancy. She was under 35, a healthy nonsmoker who only occasionally drank alcohol and had no problem giving it up while she was pregnant. She was compliant with her prenatal care, and while she considered giving birth outside the hospital, she and her husband felt that the hospital was the safest place for their first baby to be born. As a pediatrician in a small town, I was recommended to Rachel's parents by a handful of people they knew. In some respects, our community is connected by even fewer than six degrees. I had not directly met Rachel's mother, Mary Jane, but I had seen her perform with a local dance troupe. I was also connected to Rachel's dad, Tristan, as the pediatrican for members of his extended family. Both Mary Jane and Tristan are friendly, down-to-earth people who are active in their church and are close to their extended families.

Mary Jane's labor at term was not unusual in that it was not prolonged or complicated by evidence that the baby was not tolerating the contractions (otherwise known as fetal distress). She desired as few medical interventions as possible and did not ask for an epidural catheter for pain relief. Rachel was born spontaneously by vaginal delivery but was not very vigorous at birth. Still, she did not need resuscitation, and she improved with close skin-to-skin contact with her mother, as all infants do.

As Mary Jane's labor was not complicated, there was no reason for the family doctor attending to her to call me in for Rachel's birth. The family doctor, whose competence I respect and whose own child is a patient of mine (again, fewer than six degrees), called me in when Rachel was about 40 minutes old, because she started to "grunt."

Grunting respirations in a newborn can be a part of a normal transition out of the womb and into breathing air, but they also can be a sign of respiratory distress.

My initial assessment of Rachel was that she was clearly sick but that I could stabilize her and transfer her to a newborn intensive care unit, where she could receive the most appropriate care. In a short time, however, she became very unstable. Out of nowhere, the words "This baby is going to die," came out of my mouth, although it was as if it was not me who was saying them. While that may sound as though I was giving up, in reality, I became focused and organized in my task.

Rachel would be intubated and placed on a ventilator, with labs and antibiotics to follow. I inserted an intravenous catheter in Rachel's tiny hand so she could receive fluid and antibiotic therapy. Among her prenatal labs, Mary Jane had had a vaginal culture done several weeks earlier, which was negative for group B strep colonization — which can cause infection in newborns. Even though Mary Jane's pregnancy and labor history did not put Rachel at high risk for infection, there was no evidence on Rachel's physical exam that she had any anatomic or developmental abnormality to explain why she was so sick, so I was treating her for infection — in particular, for group B strep.

When an infant (or anyone else) is sick and requires significant support, the process can be simplified as A, B, C: airway, breathing, circulation. Rachel was having trouble getting air in and out and needed help. Intubating her, or placing a breathing tube in her trachea, did not help. I had no trouble seeing her vocal cords and passing an endotrachial tube through them, but when it actually came to ventilating her lungs with positive pressure, it was as though they were too stiff to inflate. I had better luck helping her breathe through a mask with positive pressure, squeezing air into her lungs from a bag. Soon, it became more and more difficult to ventilate Rachel's lungs at all, and her heart began to slow. Twice she was given chest compressions to assist her circulation, and both times she improved. But the third time her heart slowed, it did not respond to chest compressions or medication to bring the heart rate back up.

After 15 minutes of providing cardiopulmonary resuscitation, her parents requested that we cease all efforts. They felt that their daughter had fought as hard as she could.

With my own heart heavy, I turned my attention to Mary Jane and Tristan. Having been parents to a newborn daughter for only three hours, these parents reached through their unimaginable, incredible pain and sorrow to tell me that their daughter's short life should help another baby live. They did not want an autopsy performed (even though it might reveal why Rachel died), but they did want her heart valves to be recovered and donated to a baby who needed them. It was unthinkable to them to subject Rachel's little body to a postmortem examination after all it had been through in her three hours of life. Giving up the possibility of an explanation for her death was not a difficult choice for Mary Jane and Tristan.

They were sure that donating Rachel's usable heart valves was the most appropriate decision for them. I did not try to sway their decision in one direction or another, but my brain was screaming for an explanation. *Why? Why Why?* Why did a beautiful, perfect baby, born to beautiful, humble, and kind parents, die after only three hours of life?

Experiencing Rachel's life and death had an impact on me that is still difficult to articulate. It took the wind out of my sails. I kept thinking, "What did I do wrong?" And, inexplicably, "Why are Mary Jane and Tristan not blaming me for their baby's death?" The clinical review revealed no error or omission in her care, and I knew that the hospital team and I had provided appropriate and competent medical care. Still, my heart ached as if at fault for Rachel's death.

It was neither the first patient death I'd experienced nor the first infant death, but I will carry Rachel and her parents with me always.

A few months after the birth and death of their first child, Mary Jane and Tristan conceived another child. Their second baby was born, without incident, about a month after what would have been Rachel's first birthday. While Mary Jane was pregnant with this second baby, the organ and tissue donation representative informed them that Rachel's heart valves had been contaminated with group B strep bacteria. Mary Jane's 36-week culture during her first pregnancy, which could have revealed this information, might have been a false negative — or perhaps she became colonized after 36 weeks. "Why?" was finally answered, for Mary Jane and Tristan. My own screaming brain, which by now had dulled to a constant murmur of "Why?" had its answer, too. But my heart still aches and always will.

Tap

Sayantani DasGupta, MD, MPH

The tapping of a tree is not easy. The sweet sap
will not flow except under the most particular
of conditions: a freezing night followed by a
bright and sunny day. So is the delicate
balance of the sugaring season.

THE FIRST TIME I did a lumbar puncture, it felt terribly
wrong. It was two months into my internship, and I
was not yet used to the daily breaching of patients' bodies.
I was barely used to being called *doctor*.

"You've seen me do a tap," my resident said bracingly.

Not knowing yet what was coming next, I had agreed.
Yes, I had seen her do a tap — more than one. We were on
the infants' floor, and a lumbar puncture was a standard

part of the workup for the many under-two-month-old babies we saw with fevers — a diagnosis shortened on the floor to FIB, for fever in baby. FIBLETs, we called them affectionately. It was impossible to know if fevers in such young infants were due to something relatively harmless or to a more serious infection of the blood, urine, or spinal fluid. And so, along with blood and urine cultures, we tapped them.

"You've heard the phrase see one, do one, teach one?" My resident had grinned, a mother bird teaching her chick to fly. "Well, you've seen one, now it's your turn to do one."

We were in the procedure room, a tiny, windowless room at the front of the ward at a distance from the patient beds. On three of the putrid yellow walls were floor-to-ceiling metal shelves stocked with tourniquets, bandages, butterfly needles, blood tubes of all different hues, IV catheters, arm boards, tape, papooses for restraining toddlers, and, of course, the long lumbar puncture needles. At the end of the night, particularly one with a lot of admissions or procedures, the room sometimes looked as if a tornado had ripped through it — discarded packaging, dirty gloves, and gauze scattered about like fallen leaves. Despite hospital protocol, there were sometimes even used needles sticking out of the examination table — as if miniature metallic spores had grown spontaneously from the spongy cushioning. It was the intern's job to tidy the procedure room at the end of the night so that the chief residents or attendings would not witness such travesties when they came in for morning rounds.

But I was not there to clean up. Nor was I there to assist and observe — fetching equipment or folding the baby's head to its knees and holding it there in a C-shaped curve so that my resident might perform the lumbar puncture procedure. I was there to tap the baby myself. But the most important part of my job, according to my resident, came long before I even put on my sterile gloves.

"You have to be steady — delicate, but firm," she explained. In fact, she might have been describing how to advance the needle into the tender gap between the vertebrae, but she wasn't. She was telling me about the critical procedure that came before you even picked up the needle. Getting rid of the parents.

"They're worried, and you can understand that," my resident went on, her confident voice both kind and strong, "but they can't get in the way of you doing your job. It's better for them, it's better for us, and ultimately, it's better for the baby if they're not here."

Surely she was kidding. For the first time in my life, I was about to stick a needle into the back of a helpless infant to draw out the precious fluid that bathes the baby's spinal cord. And I was supposed to tell the parents of that one-month-old baby (people who were still reeling at the thought that their precious child might be seriously ill) to leave?

"Of course," my resident went on smoothly, perhaps in response to my horrified expression, "they have every right to stay. After all, it's their baby."

I nodded.

"But do these parents *really* want to see what we're going to do to their little angel? They may think they do, but do they *really*?"

I had already seen plenty of disturbing things done in that room in the name of medicine. Babies stuck and stuck again with IVs...black and blue marks on arms, legs, and, ultimately, scalps, as residents tried to find a vein that would not collapse. Screaming children held down with the weight of a full-grown intern or resident, sometimes two. I'd even heard frustrated residents whispering curses, whether to themselves, or to a torturous blood vessel, or to the struggling children upon whom they were working I was never sure.

"Mommy and Daddy don't want to cause their baby pain — they want to be waiting to rescue the baby, comfort her when the procedure is done," the resident said. "They want to be the good guys."

I nodded again, more convinced. My hands went cold at the thought of what I would soon be doing.

Before I left to speak to the parents and bring the baby to the treatment room, my teacher gave me a final piece of advice. "Look, this is the first tap you've ever done," she said matter-of-factly, fixing me squarely in her clear-eyed gaze. "Do you really want witnesses?"

That convinced me as nothing had.

"Mommy," I called cheerily as I entered the room with two beds, the twin cribs like metal cages. My heart was beating with trepidation, my palms sweating. I was expecting a confrontation. But it was all too easy.

"I'm going to take the baby now for the tests we dis-cussed." My voice sounded remarkably friendly, sunny, while my scrubs, white coat, and dangling stethoscope proclaimed my legitimacy. The young parents looked up at me with complete trust in their eyes.

As I took the tiny, swaddled bundle from her mother's arms, I heard myself say, "I promise we'll take good care of her." And they handed their firstborn child over to me without so much as a word of protest. Of course, I never even gave them any option.

This is not to say that I didn't encounter resistance from other parents who came later—I did. Weeping par-ents, anxious parents, even angry parents who hovered by the door. But none of them stayed. With increasing com-petence, I uprooted them all.

"Are you a real doctor or one of those residents?" they asked, little knowing that I was worse than a resident, a mere intern.

"I want a full-grown doctor, not one who's going to practice on my baby," they complained to the nurse, who, as a member of the club, rolled her eyes at me behind their backs.

"I'm giving you two chances and then you're out," they said. "I don't care who you have to call in the middle of the night. TWO CHANCES."

But how could they know what happened behind those closed doors?

AND SO THERE I WAS, years later, at the other end of the needle. Some kind of karmic retribution.

I was in labor with my first child and had survived 20 hours of contractions without painkillers, breathing and counting and holding my husband's hand. We had made it through lots of other long and difficult nights together — in med school, internship, residency. With him, I could make it through anything.

With the dawning of the gray morning, the OB/GYN announced that she wanted to give me pitocin to speed my labor. My water had broken the previous evening, but my body was not sufficiently dilated for the baby's birth. Seeing my distress — I had wanted nothing but a natural childbirth — my OB then suggested an epidural.

"Sometimes," she explained, "just the pain relief helps a woman dilate. And then maybe you won't need the pitocin."

I'm not sure if her logic was medically sound, but at that point, I had nothing else to go on. With the peeling away of my clothes, my privacy and my dignity had been shed — as well as my professional identity. Wrapped in a flimsy blue hospital gown, groaning with pain, my naked bottom bathed in a pool of amniotic fluid, I was nothing more or less than a patient, entirely dependent on my clinicians' care and judgment.

Whatever was left of the pediatrician in me by then only made it worse. My medical training told me we were fighting against the clock — with the possibility of ruptured membranes, there was a finite amount of time I would be allowed to labor until it became too risky. Without the protective amniotic sac, any number of infections could creep, tentacle-like, into my womb, seeding themselves in the body of my vulnerable baby. My son. My firstborn.

Since that first trembling tap, I had seen more than a few babies with perinatally acquired infections, FIBLETs who had grown horrible organisms from the blood and urine, from their spinal fluid. And, like any mother, all I wanted was a healthy baby.

So I was scheduled for an epidural.

When the anesthesiology resident arrived, the first thing he did, even before donning his gloves, was to ask my husband to leave.

The world crashed down around my ears. My plan for a natural delivery was already completely derailed. I couldn't imagine facing the epidural — a needle in my back, not unlike a lumbar puncture procedure — alone.

"I can't do this without him. I've been in labor all night," I tried to explain, my voice faint and hollow to my own ears. My teeth were chattering uncontrollably.

But my husband had already let go of my hand.

"We're doctors!" I protested, trying a different tack. "Colleagues! Can't you bend the rules for colleagues?"

But neither the anesthesia resident nor my husband was listening. They were discussing the results of some latest *New England Journal* study that had to do with both of their fields.

"Can't he please stay with me?" I begged. I was shaking from the excruciating contractions shooting from my core every two minutes. Without my husband there to hold me together, I would surely split in two.

"It's procedure," the resident explained. "It's for your own good, and ours."

And then it happened. The unimaginable. My husband actually left me. Hands deep in his pockets, he backed out of the door with a shrugged-shoulders posture that cried, "I tried my best, and after all, what else was I expected do?" Like the winter sun that vanishes abruptly below the horizon, he retreated from the room, smiling softly to no one. He was a doctor, his expression seemed to say, and he knew the rules.

I shivered. I was naked, alone, and at the mercy of a man and his needle. Never mind that in another season of my life, I would have been his superior, since even a pediatrics attending outranks an anesthesia resident. True, in the real hierarchy of the hospital, I would not be giving him orders, but I could say, as I did that day, with all the strength I could muster, "I want to speak to your attending."

With an unnecessary amount of force, he slammed down the instrument tray, wrapped like a cheap birthday present in thin blue sterile cloth. The overhead light blared down on us as if we were in a play.

"I have other patients," he hissed through gritted teeth.

I began to cry, my face contorting into ugliness. But with whatever scraps of composure I had left, I met his stare. He snorted. Naked or not, it was clear I was going to make a fuss. So he stormed into the hallway to call her.

It was cold and lonely in that anonymous labor room. Beside the hospital bed and tray table, the beeping fetal monitor, and the screen that tracked my vitals, its only attempt at decoration was an enormous black and white image of a baby's footprint on the wall directly in front of me. The magnified swirls twisted, mazelike — rings on an ancient tree. The minutes ticked by. A nurse whose name I don't remember retied my open gown and wrapped a scratchy white hospital issue blanket around me. I thanked her, and for a moment, she squeezed my shoulder.

The fetal monitor blipped on interminably.

Despite the slight respite I bought myself by having the attending paged, nothing really changed in the end. As I had probably known she would, she backed her resident's assertion that it was standard procedure not to allow spouses to be present for epidurals. Even in the case of spouses who were doctors or doctors who were patients.

"Better for everyone involved," she echoed.

So they prepped me, feeling for the bony landmarks on my pregnant body, pressing with a fingernail between my lumbar vertebrae until they left a mark, swirling the cold clammy Betadine on my curved back.

They placed a blue sterile drape with the exposed hole over my lower spine and ordered me to bend even further. The once kind nurse shoved down my neck and gripped my arms so hard she left bruises.

I shook in fear, humiliation, and a terrible loneliness. The doctors barked at me. Hadn't they warned me not to move?

Then they stuck that needle into my spine, as I had done so many times before to so many countless babies. Stripped of my connections and community — without a familiar face, a comforting voice — my very sense of selfhood dissolved such that I was no longer something solid in this world but a hole, an absence, a space drilled out of the person I once called myself.

MOTHERHOOD

Lee Savio Beers, MD

IT IS NEVER EASY TO talk about, so I will just say it: I have
had three miscarriages over the past five years. I am also,
most importantly, blessed with two healthy and beautiful
children, which means I have spent the better part of the
past few years either pregnant or nursing. While medical
school and residency were formative times, my experience
as a pediatrician has been shaped equally, if not more, by
the joys and losses I experienced in becoming a mother.

Before I had children, people always used to ask me
what it was like to be a pediatrician when I didn't have
kids of my own. "It is no problem," I would tell them, a
little bit offended. "I try to listen to families, and I think
I am fairly empathetic." And, in retrospect, I think that

was true — I was very connected to many of the families I cared for and tried to be flexible and understanding of the real-life pressures of being a parent. I also know many excellent pediatricians, for whom I have a great deal of respect, who don't have children of their own.

But I think I understand now the real meaning behind the question — it is about understanding, in a way you can understand only through experience, that feeling deep down in your gut when you are worried your child is very sick or you realize you may lose your child before you have ever gotten the chance to know him or her. My first pregnancy ended in miscarriage toward the end of the first trimester. Early ultrasounds indicated that things were not as they should be, so theoretically, I should have been prepared for the day the obstetrician told me he couldn't see a heartbeat. I was by myself — my husband, who is also a pediatrician, and I had overestimated our ability to remain clinical and detached in the face of our own pregnancy and loss. In shock and overwhelming grief, I was barely able to cancel the rest of my patients for the day and drive home. We knew that miscarriage is relatively common and that many women who have a miscarriage go on to have healthy pregnancies. However, that didn't diminish our grief for the baby or our fear that we would never deliver a healthy child.

It was almost a year before I was pregnant again, and I was terrified. I would duck into the bathroom for no reason other than to make sure I wasn't bleeding. Yet, since my first miscarriage had been diagnosed by ultrasound, without any initial cramping or bleeding, even that was not reassuring. I was feeling much more nauseated this time around, which I took as a good sign. The downside was that every time I didn't feel nauseated, I worried that something was going wrong. Thankfully, despite my worries, I went on to have a completely uncomplicated pregnancy, and I delivered a screaming baby girl at 3:00 AM on my due date.

However, even having a normal pregnancy the second time around did not completely ease my anxiety when my husband and I decided we were ready for a second child. I was calmer, to be sure, knowing that my body was capable of carrying a child to term, but I always had the knowledge at the back of my mind that it was very easy for things to go wrong. I went on to have two more miscarriages — the second one at the very end of the first trimester, after I had finally relaxed and allowed myself to believe that all was well. When I became pregnant yet again, very quickly after that last miscarriage, I essentially shut down my emotions and shuffled through the next four months, just waiting for the other shoe to drop. The bad news never came, but I wasn't able to let go of the anxiety until I was holding our eight-pound, five-ounce baby boy in my arms. I had been blessed with an uncomplicated pregnancy. I wouldn't trade my children for the world, and if we had to suffer losses to get there, in retrospect it was entirely worth it. However, as a friend said to me after my third miscarriage, it would be much easier in hard times to accept that everything was going to turn out all right if only you knew exactly when and how it was going to happen.

Just weeks after my first miscarriage, I was talking with the mother of one of my patients. I knew this mother fairly well, as I had taken many panicked phone calls from her about clinically minor concerns or illnesses. I had just finished talking with her for a fairly long time during a busy day, when she said, "Thank you, Dr. Beers, for taking the time to talk with me. I'm sorry I'm always so anxious, but I had 13 miscarriages before Emily was born — I guess I'm just still afraid something will happen to her." My stomach tightened. Thirteen miscarriages, I thought — I don't know how she handled it. I was still devastated from just one. Yet here she was with a vibrant and healthy young daughter — though I understood the look of fear in her eyes every time her daughter hit her head or spiked a fever. Thirteen times she had at least a moment of hope, and each time, she lost her baby. I could imagine how hard it still must be to believe that it wasn't going to happen again.

Several months later, before I was pregnant for the second time, I was working at one of our hospital's community clinics in the most impoverished area of Washington, D.C. A young teenager was brought to the office by her mother for very heavy vaginal bleeding. A pregnancy test quickly confirmed that she was pregnant and, based on her symptoms, probably having a miscarriage. Both she and her mother were quite scared and upset that she was losing her pregnancy. We cared for her medically and provided support and reassurance until she was able to be transferred to the emergency department. Remembering the similar experience I'd had — rushing to the emergency room in the middle of the night for uncontrollable bleeding as my first pregnancy came to a close — I felt an unexpected connection. Our lives could not have been more different. Yet through this shared experience, I was able to see her not as an irresponsible teenager who was probably better off (as some of the staff suggested) but simply as a mother experiencing a loss.

Over and over, I have had patient encounters that have reinforced my own emotions and fears. The 45-year-old first-time mother who, after struggling through infertility treatments, felt guilty because she was having a hard time adjusting to the change in lifestyle that comes with having a newborn. The young couple who woke up to discover their infant son had died overnight. The adolescent mother struggling to decide whether she should make the agonizing decision to terminate a second unwanted pregnancy. Both the fear and the experience of loss are very real to parents and affect their behavior in many subtle, and not-so-subtle, ways. I have always been aware of this but am even more attuned to it now.

Does being a mother, particularly one who has not come by it easily, make me a better pediatrician? I don't think so. Does it make me a different kind of pediatrician? It probably does. Does it change the way I experience being a pediatrician? Most definitely. It is harder to remain clinical and detached when you care for families who are suffering a loss or caring for a sick child. While I will never know exactly what my patients and their families are going through, because we all have different backgrounds and lives, I still have that feeling, deep down in my stomach, when I see them struggle. Sometimes that is probably good; through my sympathy, I can provide support and help families cope. Other times my perception of their experience is colored by my own, and it is harder to be objective or know when to pull back.

All specialties of medicine involve not just the patient but the whole family; however, pediatrics is unique in the extent to which your patient is the family. The family, whether biological or otherwise, is responsible for a child's health and well-being. The parents may have many struggles of their own and may not be well equipped to care for another, but they still love their children. It may be hard to see that love sometimes, particularly when children are abused or neglected, but I do think there is always something there. We all have a profound connection to our children, and as a pediatrician, it is my job to seek that out.

Close Calls

Perri Klass, MD

I DIDN'T REALIZE I WAS on call that night until we were at Fenway Park and the ball game was well under way. Call started at 9:00 PM, and frankly, I was lucky I even heard my beeper chirp its forlorn, reproachful, you-have-a-page-you-haven't-looked-at alert. But around 9:02, I found myself taking leave of my family and making people stand up all along the row of seats so I could get out and look for someplace reasonably quiet to take my call. And thinking, resentfully, "Damn it, am I actually on *call* tonight? Can't a person even go to a Red Sox game in peace?"

Of course, there *is* no reasonably quiet place at Fenway during a game. I found myself on an open-air stairway cantilevered out over the street — you could tell from the scent that people went there to sneak cigarettes. It was early in the 2005 season, my last full summer in Boston, and the Red Sox roster was full of uncertainties. Yes, there was the delirious, improbable high after the 2004 World Series championship, but there were also lots of questions about the pitching rotation, and things were looking dicey for both Curt Schilling, the past season's star of a starting pitcher, and Keith Foulke, the past season's rock-solid, dependable closer.

The first call was pretty routine. Yes, you can give her the amoxicillin and the ibuprofen together. No, you don't give a child fever medicine according to age, you give it according to weight. The crowd was screaming. I apologized for the noise, asked the child's weight, converted pounds to kilos in my head, and verified the ibuprofen dose.

I made my way back to my seat. Fenway Park is a glorious historic shrine to baseball, but there isn't a lot of room between the rows of seats. And though a certain amount of coming and going is de rigueur during a ball game, what with trips to buy beer and trips to buy hot dogs, I felt sure that the people in my row could tell that I was not disturbing them for any proper ballpark business. My son greeted me and updated me on the progress of the game.

Baseball has been used as a metaphor for everything in the world. Baseball is theater; baseball is war; baseball is life. And medicine is full of sports metaphors. As a medical student doing my first rotation on the internal medicine wards, I struggled to master the medico-base-ball jargon, as if that would reflect my clinical knowledge. How many hits did your team get last night? You're kidding — a no-hitter? Hey, did you hear that? Team A had a no-hitter!

But sitting at Fenway Park and waiting for the answering service to page me, I couldn't extend the metaphor in any trenchant way. I didn't think about the way life deals out balls and strikes to parents as they struggle from inning to inning, or any such nonsense. I was angry at myself for not having checked the call schedule; I could have switched evenings with someone else. I was irritated with my job, which seemed regularly to reach out of right and reasonable boundaries to claim other little pieces of my life — there I was at Fenway Park on a nice spring evening with my family, and instead of sitting with them and cheering, I was stuck answering calls. Now that I knew I was on call, I had to keep my beeper somewhere where I would be sure to hear it. In a decisive ballpark fashion statement, I clipped it to the neck of my shirt, right up near my ears. And then I prayed silently that it would be a quiet night — and, since all prayers in Fenway Park are required to end this way, that the Red Sox would hold it together and win the game.

The beeper went off again. I considered returning the page from my seat. After all, people do talk on their cell phones during ball games — all around me, I could hear people announcing their location to friends at home ("Yeah, I'm at Fenway Park!") or trying to locate friends in the park ("Meet me near the place where they sell beer — no, not that one, the other one!"). But I couldn't imagine being on the phone with a patient's mother surrounded by this much noise — and sure enough, the umpire made an obviously ridiculous call right around then, the noise level rose dramatically, and not all the language being used would have been, shall we say, appropriate in a pediatric context.

So I excused myself back out of the row, making everyone stand up once again, and found my spot on the stairway. Another pretty routine call, a baby with a bad cold. Lots of coughing, lots of mucus, not eating as well as usual, but no fever, no wheezing — not so sick, by the sound of it. I talked about humidifiers and fever control and what to watch for. I apologized for all the background noise.

It was getting late in the game, toward 10:00. They had stopped selling beer. The Red Sox were not playing brilliantly. Plenty of fans had left, and there were empty seats in our section, so I sat in one right on the aisle so I could respond to pages more easily. I felt a little more relaxed, no longer resenting my job so much — in fact, it seemed to me that the job was part of what connected me to Boston: here I was in this civic shrine, cheering on the home team, while responding to questions from worried parents all over the city. I felt established and appropriately involved — and hopeful that the Red Sox might win the game for me. And my beeper went off.

And that time, I got it — the page that you don't want as an on-call pediatrician, let alone from a parent who doesn't speak English very clearly, let alone when you're stuck in a noisy public place. Picture me, standing out there on the stairs, yelling into my cell phone: *How* high is his fever? *How* much temperature? *How* many *times* did he throw up? *What* are you saying about his neck? Does he have *pain* in his neck? Is it stiff? His *neck*, I'm asking you if it's *stiff.* Does it hurt? Pain? Does he have any pain there in his *neck?* But the poor father on the other end didn't really have the vocabulary for this, or maybe it was hard to hear me. All I could tell for sure was that there was a child with fever, and something wrong with his neck, and he kept vomiting.

"Go to the emergency room!" I shouted, as the crowd roared its approval of a well-pitched strike — or maybe of a clumsily thrown ball; I no longer knew which team was batting. I had lost track. "You have to take the baby to the hospital! To the emergency room!"

The father said something I couldn't quite make out — I think he was asking me if he could just give the child Tylenol to bring the fever down.

"Take him to the emergency room — to the hospital!" I bellowed. "He might be very sick! This is very important!"

Another crowd roar for a strike or a ball — we were getting to that tense end-of-game zone where you react to every pitch. And all I could imagine was disaster — the kid had bacterial meningitis, I was sure of it. The worried parents, summoning every shred of their English, had called the health center and struggled heroically to communicate with the answering service, and then the doctor called back and it sounded like she was in some crazy place, surrounded by a screaming mob, so much noise, so hard to understand her. There was no rule against taking calls from Fenway Park, yet in that moment I could envision a front-page scandal: the heedless doctor disporting herself at the ball game, the worried parents watching their child get sicker and sicker.

"TAKE HIM TO THE HOSPITAL!" I roared. "RIGHT NOW! TO THE HOSPITAL!"

Okay, the father said. Okay, they would do it.

I called in an expect, made my way off the staircase, and sank down again into the aisle seat. Yes, please, they should take him to the emergency room, they should listen to me. No, they shouldn't decide just to give him some fever medicine instead. And at the ER, he should please not have meningitis. And all should be well — and could the Red Sox please just hold it together long enough to win the stupid game?

After that, my beeper was quiet. The game was almost over, and the Red Sox were clinging to a lead. They put Keith Foulke in to close — the man who had pitched the final victorious inning of the last game of the 2004 World Series, who had fielded the last out, flipping the ball to first base to end the game. I was watching carefully now, though I was still aware of my beeper. If the Red Sox win, I thought, it will be okay: I will call the ER, and they'll tell me the child was fine, no meningitis, maybe a minor torticollis. If the Red Sox win, there will be no white cells in the boy's cerebrospinal fluid (CSF). I was leaning forward, counting every pitch along with the crowd. We were loyal to Foulke but worried. In fact, he had a rocky time, and he didn't close it easily, but the Red Sox won, and we all applauded and shuffled our way out of Fenway Park, and I thought that at least now I would be able to answer any other calls in peace.

Needless to say, once I got out of the ballpark, the calls stopped. I did call the ER, and they told me the child had looked kind of sick but had revived significantly after being given antipyretics and a few glasses of juice. Yes, they had done the lumbar puncture, because the history was suggestive of meningitis, but they hadn't been surprised that the tap was negative. It really didn't look like meningitis.

"It was hard to tell, over the phone," I said. "You know how it is."

I would like to be able to offer you a profound metaphorical connection between baseball and medicine. I would like to be able to say that taking calls from the ballpark taught me something other than the obvious lesson that there are moments when patients' lives and doctors' lives intersect in a way not quite like what you read in the medical textbooks — like on that night when I really did feel sure for a little while that if the Red Sox hung on to the lead and won the game, the child's CSF would be clear and, thanks to my many years of medical training, my prediction turned out to be correct. But I had no easy lesson to learn, no easy profundity to teach — I remembered being on call at Fenway, even though I never let it happen again.

I thought about that night again this past May, when Jon Lester pitched his no-hitter for the Red Sox against the Royals. There he was, 24 years old, and as he made his way into the seventh inning, the radio announcers started discussing the no-hitter with every out, which makes me nervous, because you really aren't supposed to mention that there's a no-hitter in progress. They also had to remind us, at least once an inning, that Lester had survived cancer two years before and had come back to pitch in the final game of the 2007 World Series after finishing treatment for lymphoma — and now here he was, the cancer survivor, pitching a no-hitter.

I couldn't listen to the eighth inning. If it fell apart in the eighth, I didn't want to know about it. But I came back for the ninth — who could stay away? Lester walked the first batter but got the second to ground out. And while I was out of the room for the eighth, I had thought about that on-call night at Fenway three years ago and about conflating the baseball gods and the medical gods, and I wondered whether there actually was some parallel to be drawn.

I thought about statistics and probabilities — what was the chance that that child really had bacterial meningitis, in this age of vaccination against Hib and pneumococcus? What are the odds that a child's fever represents bacterial meningitis? You know the answer: it's unlikely, but if it's your child, your patient, it's 100 percent. What's the five-year survival rate for any particular kind of cancer? What's the next batter's batting average? What's his lifetime record against left-handed pitchers? Baseball is, after all, a game of statistics — knowing the statistics, defying the statistics, celebrating the statistics. And the odds of a no-hitter are small indeed, even for great and experienced pitchers.

There was definitely something to be learned here, about baseball, about medicine, I thought, as Lester got the second out in the ninth. Maybe something about how it's not only about the odds of survival — and sometimes about beating those odds — but also about how surviving means open odds on all the other likely and unlikely things you can do with the rest of your life. And Jon Lester struck out the last batter in the ninth, and the announcers let us know: one for the record books.

ACKNOWLEDGMENT OF PERMISSIONS

"Jazmine" is excerpted from *Almost Home* by Christine Gleason and is used with the permission of the author and Kaplan Publishing.

"Shifting Sands" first appeared in the *New England Journal of Medicine* in Volume 352, Number 1 (January 2005). It is reprinted with the permission of Perri Klass and the publisher.

"There's a Bug in Your Head" first appeared in the *Hastings Center Report* in Volume 36, Number 3 (May–June 2006). It is reprinted with the permission of the author and the publisher.

"Close Calls" first appeared in the *New England Journal of Medicine* in Volume 359, Number 10 (September 2008). It is reprinted with the permission of Perri Klass and the publisher.

Reader's Guide

1. In William Borkowsky's story, "Path to Pediatrics," he describes the care and thought processes that went into choosing pediatrics as a specialty. As you chose your own path, how did your experience compare to his? What factors did you consider?

2. In "My Mentor Was a Swine," Stacy Beller Stryer reveals how an embarrassing moment (and ultimately, being able to laugh about it) helped her overcome her fears and taught her some lifelong skills. Thinking about your own training experiences, which moments stand out as crucial, even though they were difficult and/or humbling at the time?

3. Suzanne Dixon's story, "Who's Responsible Here?", explores what responsibility means, both in individual cultures and in a larger human sense. She describes her feelings of guilt over the death of a child, even though she worked to treat the baby to the best of her

abilities. Have you ever felt responsible for a situation (medical or otherwise) that was out of your control? If so, how did you address those feelings of blame?

4. Also, what is the doctor's role in correcting cultural ideas or assumptions that might interfere with a medical explanation? How should a doctor address and respect these kinds of differences, while offering a scientific perspective?

5. In "Cuba," Lee Savio Beers works to overcome insufficient resources and isolation to give her patients the best possible care. Describe a situation where you've had to speak up to get the resources you need or had to think creatively to get out of danger.

6. Several of the stories, particularly "Paula's Story" by Mariana Glusman and "The Gift of Sight" by Diego Chaves-Gnecco, reflect on the challenges of overcoming language and cultural barriers to give the best possible care to kids. What kinds of cultural differences have you faced with your own patients? How did you approach them? Did you come away from the situation with a better understanding of different sets of values and experiences?

7. In "Tap" by Sayantani DasGupta, the author draws parallels between her experience as the doctor administering a procedure and her subsequent experience

as the patient receiving a similar procedure. Discuss a situation where a personal event gave you a better understanding of your professional life.

8. Similarly, in "Motherhood," Lee Savio Beers reflects on the relationship between being a parent and being a pediatrician. How do you think one role would impact the other?

9. "Close Calls" by Perri Klass illustrates that a pediatrician's work is never done, particularly when one is on call. Can you think of a situation where you had to make personal sacrifices to care for patients?

About the Editor

PERRI KLASS, MD, is a professor of journalism and pediatrics at New York University School of Medicine. She attended Harvard Medical School and completed her residency in pediatrics at Children's Hospital Boston. She is the medical director of the Reach Out and Read program, a national pediatric literacy program that works through health care providers to encourage early literacy and reading aloud to young children.

Dr. Klass is an extensively published author who has published two well-known books about her own medical training, *A Not Entirely Benign Procedure: Four Years as a Medical Student* and *Baby Doctor: A Pediatrician's Training*. Her most recent book about the medical field is *Treatment Kind and Fair: Letters to a Young Doctor*.

She is also the author of four novels, most recently *The Mercy Rule*; the coauthor of a memoir, *Every Mother Is a Daughter: The Neverending Quest for Success, Inner Peace, and a Really Clean Kitchen*, written with her mother, Sheila Solomon Klass; and coauthor of *Quirky Kids: Understanding and Helping Your Child Who Doesn't Fit In*, written with Dr. Eileen Costello. She writes regularly for the *New York Times* and for many other newspapers and magazines, including *Parenting, Diversion*, and *Knitters*.

ABOUT THE
CONTRIBUTORS

DR. LEE SAVIO BEERS, MD, is an assistant professor of pediatrics at Children's National Medical Center and The George Washington University Medical Center. She is the director of the Healthy Generations Program, a "teen-tot" program providing comprehensive medical care, case management, and mental health services to adolescent parents and their children. Dr. Beers received a bachelor of science degree from The College of William and Mary and her medical degree from Emory University School of Medicine. She completed a pediatric residency at Naval Medical Center Portsmouth. Before coming to Children's Hospital, she worked as a general pediatrician at Naval Hospital Guantánamo Bay in Cuba and National Naval Medical Center in Bethesda, Maryland. She is a graduate of the George Washington University Graduate School of Education and Human Development Master Teacher Certificate in Medical Education Program.

Dr. Beers has held numerous leadership positions in the American Academy of Pediatrics and is currently a member of the National Committee on Residency Scholarships. She is on the editorial board and writes a monthly column entitled "On the Learning Curve" for *Pediatric News*. Her professional and research interests include adolescent pregnancy and parenting, including fathers; medical education; and the prevention of child abuse and neglect. She has both published and given numerous local and national presentations on these topics.

WILLIAM BORKOWSKY, MD, is a professor of pediatrics at New York University.

DIEGO CHAVES-GNECCO, MD, MPH, is an assistant professor of pediatrics at the University of Pittsburgh School of Medicine. He obtained his title as a medical doctor from Pontificia Universidad Javeriana in Bogotá, Colombia. He completed his residency in Pediatrics in Colombia between 1995 and 1998 at Hospital Universitario San Ignacio, Clínicas Infantiles Cafám y Colsubsidio, serving as chief of residents during his last year. In 1998, Dr. Chaves-Gnecco moved to Pittsburgh as a visiting instructor at the University of Pittsburgh, School of Medicine–Center for Clinical Pharmacology, where he worked until 2002. He obtained a master's degree in Public Health from the University of Pittsburgh Graduate School of Public Health in 2000. He completed his residency in pediatrics in the United States at Children's Hospital of Pittsburgh of UPMC between 2002 and 2005. He also completed a fellowship in developmental-behavioral pediatrics at the same institution between 2005 and 2008. In the summer of 2002, Dr. Chaves-Gnecco created the first pediatric bilingual-bicultural clinic in southwestern Pennsylvania, Salud Para Niños (Health for Children). Dr. Chaves-Gnecco has been honored with several recognitions of his work and of his services to the community.

EILEEN COSTELLO, MD, is a primary care pediatrician in Boston. She trained at Boston City Hospital and Children's Hospital Medical Center in Boston, and has practiced in urban neighborhood health centers in Boston for 19 years. She is the co-author of *Quirky Kids: Understanding and Helping Your Child Who Doesn't Fit In — When to Worry and When Not to Worry* (2003, Ballantine Books). Her particular interests in pediatrics include caring for children on the autism spectrum, the care of newborns and their families, and working with children with mental illness.

SAYANTANI DASGUPTA, MD MPH, is assistant professor of clinical pediatrics and core faculty in the Program in Narrative Medicine at Columbia University. She also teaches courses in illness narratives and narrative genetics at Sarah Lawrence College, where she is a prose instructor in their Writing the Medical Experience summer seminar. She is the coauthor of *The Demon Slayers and Other Stories: Bengali Folktales*; the author of a memoir about her education at Johns Hopkins Medical School, *Her Own Medicine: A Woman's Journey from Student to Doctor*; and coeditor of an independent publishing award-winning collection of women's illness narratives, *Stories of Illness and Healing: Women Write Their Bodies.* She is an associate editor of the journal *Literature and Medicine*, and her writing has been published in a variety of locations, including *JAMA, Pediatrics*, the *Hastings Center Report*, and the *Journal of Medical Humanities.*

SUZANNE DIXON, MD, MPH, is a developmental and behavioral pediatrician now practicing and doing advocacy work in Montana. She is the editor of the *Journal of Developmental and Behavioral Pediatrics* and the author/ editor of the pediatric textbook *Encounters with Children: Pediatric Behavior and Development*, now in its fourth edition. She is a professor emerita from the University of California, San Diego, and holds a clinical professorship from the University of Washington. She has done research, advocacy, and program development work concerning perinatal care, parenting, and child development all around the world.

CHRISTINE GLEASON, MD, grew up in Rochester, New York. She attended Brown University and received her medical degree from the University of Rochester. Dr. Gleason did her pediatric residency training in Cleveland and her neonatology fellowship training in San Francisco. Her first job as a full-fledged neonatologist was at John

Hopkins Hospital, where she became chief of neonatology. She moved to Seattle in 1997 as chief of neonatology and professor of pediatrics at the University of Washington and Seattle Children's Hospital. She lives in Seattle with her husband, three daughters, and a golden retriever named Molly.

MARIANA GLUSMAN, MD, is an assistant professor of pediatrics at Northwestern University. She received her undergraduate degree at Brown University and her medical degree at the University of Chicago's Pritzker School of Medicine. She completed her pediatric residency at Children's Memorial Hospital in 1996, and has been a pediatrician at the Children's Uptown Clinic since then. Her areas of interest include literacy promotion in the pediatric setting, health literacy, health disparities, working with Latino families, improving links between pediatricians and schools, and language development. Dr. Glusman has been the medical director for Reach Out and Read of Illinois since 2006. She is working on multiple initiatives to expand the program throughout the state, to form closer links with the library system, to train providers on adult health literacy and to improve outreach to Latino families. Dr. Glusman lives in Chicago with her husband and three children.

RACHEL H. KOWALSKI, MD, graduated from Brown University in 1997 with a BA in Comparative Literature. She studied medicine at Tufts University School of Medicine, where she also received her master's in Public Health. She contributes regularly to *Tufts Medicine* magazine. Dr. Kowalski also writes fiction and was a guest artist at New York Mills Cultural Center in 2002. She completed a pediatric residency and emergency medicine fellowship in New York City. She lives in New York with her husband and daughter.

PATRICK MCDONALD, MD, MHSC, FRCSC, is associate professor of neurosurgery at the University of Manitoba and the director of pediatric neurosurgery at Winnipeg Children's Hospital in Winnipeg, Manitoba, Canada. He is a research associate at the University of Manitoba's Centre for Professional and Applied Ethics.

DIPESH NAVSARIA, MD, MPH, MSLIS, is a third-year pediatric resident in the Midwest. Born in the United Kingdom and raised in New York city, his "scenic route" to his career included a master's degree in public health, time as a physician assistant, and a hiatus in the midst of medical school to obtain a master's degree in Library and Information Science while working as a children's librarian. He plans to combine community pediatrics with teaching, advocacy and promoting early childhood literacy awareness.

JOY MARASCO NEYHART, DO, FAAP, is a primary care pediatrician practicing in Juneau, Alaska. She attended the University of Medicine and Dentistry of New Jersey and received her pediatric training at the Children's Hospital of New Jersey at Newark-Beth Israel Medical Center. She is the physician consultant to the Juneau School District and serves on the board of directors for the nonprofit Juneau Montessori School. Her main areas of interest in primary care pediatrics are breast-feeding advocacy and supporting families through education and preventative health care.

HUY QUANG NGUYEN, MD, was born in Thu Duc, Vietnam, in 1974. He immigrated with his family to the United States in 1975. After medical school at Harvard, he trained in pediatrics at the University of Washington in Seattle. Dr. Nguyen is on staff at Boston Medical Center and has practiced pediatrics at the Dorchester House, a community health center in Boston, for five years. He is married with two sons and lives in the Boston area.

MICHAEL PATRICK, MD, is a board-certified pediatrician and Fellow of the American Academy of Pediatrics. He is also host and producer of *PediaCast*, an award-winning online audio program featuring news parents can use, answers to listener questions, and interviews with pediatric specialists and parenting experts. Michael attended The Ohio State University College of Medicine and spent ten years caring for kids in Springfield, Ohio, before moving south in search of warmth and sunshine. He now lives in central Florida with his wife, Karen, and their two children, KT and Nick.

STACY BELLER STRYER, MD, graduated from Yale University School of Medicine and completed her residency in pediatrics at Children's Hospital of Northern California. She and her late husband, an internist, then spent three years working on the Navajo reservation in Kayenta, Arizona. They had many wonderful adventures on the "rez," including the birth of their first daughter. Dr. Stryer currently works in private practice in Rockville, Maryland. She is also a writer, speaker, consultant, and blogger. She worked for several years for Revolution Health and currently consults for getbetterhealth.com. Dr. Stryer loves spending time with her two daughters, especially when it involves hiking, camping, skiing, or traveling.

BRYAN VARTABEDIAN, MD, is an assistant professor of pediatrics at Baylor College of Medicine in Houston, Texas, and attending physician at Texas Children's Hospital. He is the author of *Colic Solved – The Essential Guide to Infant Reflux and the Care of Your Crying, Difficult-to-Soothe Baby* (Ballantine/Random House, 2007) and *First Foods* (St. Martin's Press, 2001). He lives with his wife and two children in The Woodlands, Texas.

ALENKA ZEMAN, MD, is Chief Resident in pediatrics at Massachusetts General Hospital for Children. She grew up in Winchester, Massachusetts, and obtained her undergraduate degree at Brown University in biology. After graduation, she was awarded an Arnold Fellowship and spent a year working at a pediatric hospital in

Prague, Czech Republic. She traveled to California to attend medical school at Stanford University. Next year, she looks forward to pursuing a career in primary care in the Boston area.

SHARE YOUR STORIES WITH KAPLAN PUBLISHING

KAPLAN PUBLISHING, a leading educational resource for doctors, would like to feature your story in an upcoming anthology in the *Kaplan Voices: Doctors* series. Please share the stories behind the relationships, the experiences, and the issues you've encountered in your medical career—whether you work in a bustling hospital, a rural clinic, private practice, or anywhere in between.

Entertaining and educational, inspirational and practical, each *Kaplan Voices: Doctors* anthology features true, first-person stories written by doctors themselves, revealing the person behind the white coat.

For writers' guidelines or more information, please contact Kaplan Publishing by email at *kaplanvoicesdoctors@gmail.com*, or write to us at:

Kaplan Voices: Doctors editor
Kaplan Publishing
1 Liberty Plaza, 24th Floor
New York, NY 10006